FIND GOOD
HABITS

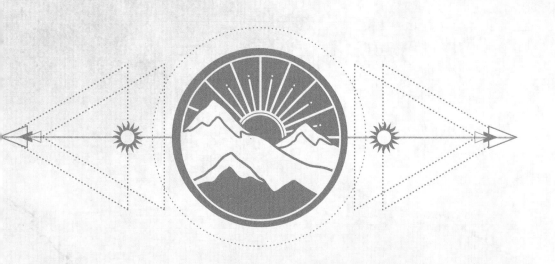

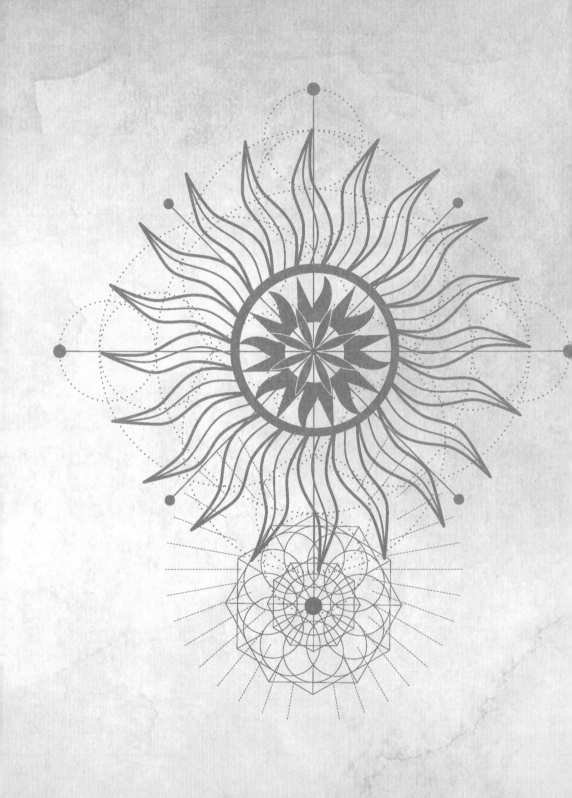

FIND GOOD
HABITS

A WORKBOOK *for* DAILY GROWTH

JAIME ZUCKERMAN, PSY.D.

WELLFLEET
PRESS

CONTENTS

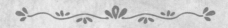

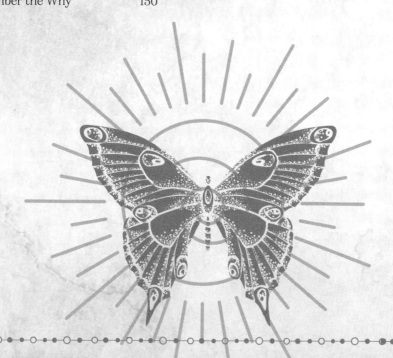

INTRODUCTION

"Why do I keep dating the same type of person?"

"Why do people routinely take advantage of me?"

"Why do I keep getting myself stuck in the same situation?"

These are the questions I frequently hear from my patients, which are the source of much of their distress, anger, and anxiety. People come to therapy because they feel stuck: stuck in their jobs, in their relationships, and just in life in general. What once worked for them is no longer effective. They feel unfulfilled and less motivated, yet they are unable to articulate why. It's this "why" that becomes the focus of therapy. I help people understand why they continue to put themselves in the same unhealthy situations, show them how to change the patterns and habits that keep them stuck, and how to maintain new behaviors so that they can live a more fulfilled and productive life.

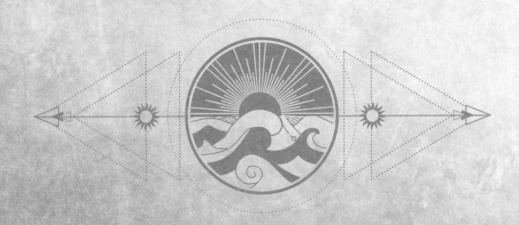

What Is
A HABIT?

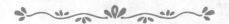

A habit can be any behavior you do that is automatic; something you do that you may not even be aware of while it's happening. It's a behavior that has become second nature. And while it may not have started out that way, it has become habitual over time. An example of a daily habit could be something as simple as biting your nails when you are nervous, overeating when you are stressed, expressing gratitude daily, or even checking your phone and mindlessly scrolling through social media. It's only when habit-type behaviors are brought into your awareness that you are able to notice them in the moment. This is often initiated by some type of external trigger. For example, maybe while biting your nails during an argument with a friend you bite too hard and it hurts. That instant feeling of pain almost shocks you out of your habitual nail-biting, allowing you to notice the behavior at the time. Or, maybe while out to dinner on a date you are habitually scrolling through your phone looking at social media posts. The waitress comes over to your table, asks

you for your drink order, which then grabs your attention away from the picture of your old college roommate's new puppy, and redirects you to the present moment. It's in this moment that behavior changes can be made. As I always like to say when working with patients, "the power is in the pause."

So, where do these habits come from? How are they formed? If we think about how our worlds were shaped throughout our upbringing, we were exposed to numerous behavior patterns by those within our immediate environments. We learned, and subsequently modeled, ways of interacting with the world around us and how to view ourselves in relation to others. As a child, we internalize the interaction styles and self-narratives given to us, which, over time, become patterns.

Simply put, a pattern is a behavior that sticks with time. In fact, patterns are all around us, not just in our behaviors. Patterns are found in nature, mathematics, language—even in the creation of city blocks. They are what make our world more predictable; a way to achieve consistency out of chaos and uncertainty. Patterns will generally have more of a familiar quality to them. This is because they are based upon the longstanding beliefs we have about ourselves stemming from childhood. They are predictable and pervasive interaction styles that we apply within ourselves and our relationships; themes we continuously fall back on without giving it much thought. It is these behavior patterns that lead to the creation of habits. As our patterns become more familiar over our lifetime, and our behaviors more frequent, habits are formed.

The Role OUR BRAINS PLAY

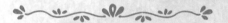

Human beings are creatures of habit. We crave predictability, structure, and routine. We like to know what is coming next. Patterns and habits do just this. They offer a guideline, a rulebook of sorts, which allows our brain to deal with other things in our environment that require our attention. For example, imagine driving a car for the first time and paying attention to every single component necessary to operate it effectively. We would have significantly fewer attentional resources to concentrate on anything else, such as other cars, stop signs, and road conditions. This is exactly why we would first practice in an empty parking lot and not a busy highway during rush hour traffic. The reduction of surrounding stimuli and distraction would be necessary to focus on the task at hand. Habits allow us to do things with little cognitive effort so that we can focus on new information or unexpected problems.

How Do Habits and Patterns
HELP US?

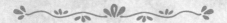

Patterns and habits both make our world more predictable and manageable. They help us to feel safe, allow us to think fast in a crisis, enable us to plan, and guide us on how to respond in social situations. They make our day-to-day lives easier and make us more productive.

Think of them of as our daily playbook, our "how-to" guide for the world around us. Even at its most basic level, a pattern or habit can tell us what comes next. For example, think of a traffic light. You are driving in your car and up ahead you see the light is yellow. As you approach, you begin to slow down, knowing that it will soon turn red, requiring you to stop until it turns green. How do you know this to be the case? You can predict the flow of the traffic light because you have experienced it many times before. Establishing, maintaining, and, when needed, adjusting patterns and habits are an integral part of our lives.

The Role
OF AVOIDANCE

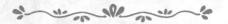

Avoidance is one of the main ingredients when it comes to unhealthy patterns and habits. It's the avoidance of our own anxiety, fear, anger, and insecurity that often leads to the development and maintenance of unhealthy behaviors. In an effort to not feel or think negative thoughts and feelings in the moment, we find ways to escape them.

The problem with this strategy is twofold. First, it only offers a temporary relief. Second, the behaviors that we commonly use to avoid our discomfort are often unhealthy. For example, using substances to avoid emotional pain, procrastinating on a project because of fear of failure, or not engaging in social interactions because you are fearful of being judged. While these behaviors may temporarily give you a sigh of relief, they actually make your angst larger and more debilitating. The temporary escape, however, sets the foundation for unhealthy pattern and habit development and maintenance. Because we crave that instant relief, we are more inclined to repeat these behaviors.

Can They
HURT US?

While patterns and habits clearly help us navigate our world, sometimes our ability to alter, modify, and change aspects of them may not be working well. The more flexible we are with our behavior, the more adaptable we become to our environments. It's when we are unwilling to shift and change our habits and patterns that they can become unhealthy.

During childhood, we develop certain patterns to help us navigate our world and our upbringing. Typically, these patterns come from modeling those of our caregivers; we repeat what we see. It's also common to develop patterns that are opposite to those of our caregivers. A child raised in a toxic family environment that may include abuse, neglect, or parental substance abuse will form patterns of behavior that help them survive. While these patterns may be effective during one's upbringing, they lose their functionality as life changes over time. In other words, what was once an effective pattern is no longer healthy. If our patterns don't adapt, neither will we. We become higher risk for anxiety, depression, substance abuse, and even physical illness.

Maintaining behavior patterns that are no longer effective also impacts the way we view ourselves within all types of relationships, including parenting, marriage, dating, and work. For example, if you were taught growing up that it is selfish or rude to focus on your own needs, you may become something of a people pleaser as an adult, gravitating toward those whose needs routinely take precedence over your own. Alternatively, internalizing the message that your needs were irrelevant as a child may lead you to project that view onto others, making your own needs the focal point of your relationships at the expense of others. The good news, however, is that regardless of age, how long you have had a particular habit, or how unhealthy that habit is, behavior change is possible by systematically integrating tiny, incremental changes throughout your day.

The Problem with
INCONSISTENCY

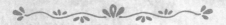

What do you think would happen if habits and patterns did not exist? If there was no predicable order of events or behaviors? With no ability to predict what comes next, we would feel extremely overwhelmed, anxious, and out of control.

When we make the commitment to change our habits and patterns, it's essential to start very small and gradually introduce additional behaviors. While the ultimate goal is for these baby steps to eventually become habitual and automatic, the most important aspect is consistency. It is better to remain consistent with a small step than to be inconsistent with bigger steps. Why is this the case? Because inconsistency in behavior change creates what's known as an intermittent reinforcement schedule. This behavior schedule is the basis of addictive behaviors such as gambling and drug addiction. These intermittent spurts of dopamine, our feel-good chemical, makes such behaviors addictive in nature. When we never know what we are going to get, it creates feelings of uncertainty, a loss of control, and heightened stress and anxiety.

This inconsistent predictability is also a factor in why people get trapped in the cycle of toxic relationships. When our significant others, friends, and family are consistent in their attention and responsiveness towards us, the relationship is viewed as dependable, predictable, and safe. It leaves very little room for ambiguity and uncertainty. You know exactly where you stand and what you can expect from them. However, when they appear hot and cold for no apparent reason or randomly disappear without warning, it can leave you feeling confused and anxious. We have all heard the saying, "walking on eggshells." This notion comes from the idea that in inconsistent relationships, we never know what we are going to get. We are constantly monitoring our behaviors, our words, and our emotions in an effort to gain some sense of consistency. Sometimes we are comforted, other times our feelings are dismissed. There is no predictability. This is intermittent reinforcement.

When applied to relationships, intermittent reinforcement creates a toxic cycle that is extremely difficult to break. What does this look like? Repeated breaking up and getting back together, explosive arguments, physical and emotional abuse, and co-dependency. The unpredictability of these dynamics creates an addictive-like quality that becomes extremely difficult to break, causing intense relationship anxiety.

What Happens When We CHANGE OUR HABITS AND PATTERNS?

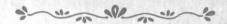

As you go through behavior-change processes, it's important to recognize that although your new behaviors may be healthier, they will likely feel uncomfortable at first. Habits are undoubtedly hard to break, and as we give up familiar behaviors, we are often faced with underlying uncomfortable feelings and thoughts. Changing longstanding behaviors can be scary. We often hold onto unhealthy habits and patterns, because by doing so we trick ourselves into thinking we are in control. Many toxic behaviors allow for us to avoid things we don't want to feel or think about in our day-to-day. This is especially true when these behaviors have been used to avoid negative emotions over a lifetime (such as drinking, or people pleasing). We know on some level that if we let go of this familiarity, we will need to face uncertainty and the discomfort associated with healthy behavior change. A rule of thumb I like

to use with my patients is: "If it feels uncomfortable at first, it's probably the healthier choice."

Interestingly, one of the more difficult things about changing patterns and habits is the impact it has on the people around us. Not only are patterns and habits part of our daily routine, but others become comfortable with them as well. For example, people who are notorious people pleasers frequently say "yes" despite being overwhelmed, keep their opinions to themselves for fear of being disliked, and often put their needs second to avoid appearing selfish. The people they surround themselves with have become accustomed to this pattern. They may inadvertently take advantage of the people-pleasing pattern, assuming this person will always be available to them. So, what happens when a people pleaser begins to change their patterns by setting boundaries and learning how to say "no?" It throws everyone else off-kilter. The dynamics between their family, friends, and coworkers become uncomfortable. And, because we are very much creatures of habit, it's not uncommon for those in the system to push back against any new pattern in an effort to restore the status quo, even if it's unhealthy. So, what might this look like in the above example? A friend might tell the people pleaser that they are being selfish, or that they are acting "different." To avoid feeling bad, the people pleaser may resort back to their original pattern, therefore restoring the dynamic to its original (and familiar) position.

The Impact on Our
MENTAL HEALTH

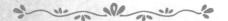

Behavior plays an extremely important role in our emotional well-being. Mood and anxiety disorders are often the result of maladaptive behaviors that have been in place for years. As mentioned previously, we develop behavioral patterns during our childhood that worked for us. These allowed us to navigate our environments as best we could, but as we develop into adulthood and our environments change, our patterns need to shift as well. In other words, our patterns must go with the flow. If we do not adjust our patterns to fit with our current context, they may no longer work for us, and instead we create unhealthy habits.

This can keep people stuck in unhealthy relationships, unfulfilling jobs, toxic friendships, and difficult life stages. Staying in these dysfunctional dynamics perpetuates toxic patterns and habits, taking a significant toll on mental health. Symptoms of depression and anxiety can develop, leading to even more unhealthy behaviors, such as isolation and substance use, as well as feelings of hopelessness and decreased self-worth.

Why then do people choose to repeat unhealthy patterns and habits? Because they are familiar, comfortable, and easy. Moreover, many people have difficulty seeing how their unhealthy behavior choices may be contributing to their current circumstances. And why would they? These are patterns that, at one point, worked quite well. It is only through identifying our habits and patterns, their origins, and the functions they serve, that we can begin to make healthy and lasting changes in our lives.

By slowly and strategically implementing healthy habits into our day, we begin to develop healthier patterns. We surround ourselves with like-minded people who support our new changes, we improve our overall mental and physical well-being, and we live longer, more fulfilled lives.

How Do We
CHANGE THEM?

It is possible to change patterns and habits, even if their origins date back to childhood. They are typically learned behaviors and therefore can be "unlearned." The first step in the change process is acknowledging that things in your life are not working well, although you may not yet understand why. Many of my patients will initially come to therapy because they are unhappy in their relationships, are experiencing a worsening of family relationships, or are unfulfilled in their careers. And while most have made considerable effort to improve their situations, things just don't seem to change. In fact, they appear to be getting worse.

A critical component of this change process is to gain awareness of how patterns or habits negatively impact someone's life. Think of patterns as a lifestyle, and in order to change or modify them, a lifestyle shift must take place. It is important to remember that not all patterns and habits are bad. In fact, many are healthy and may require only a slight adjustment—or none at all. Understanding this can help increase motivation to change and give a person the confidence that they already are capable of engaging in healthy behaviors.

Once healthy and unhealthy behaviors have been identified, alternative steps are suggested that will result in healthier choices and relationships. It is key to start small. In fact, you want to start as tiny as possible. I like to tell my patients to start "insultingly small." When people commit to change a habit or longstanding pattern, they may initially feel highly motivated and compelled to make big changes all at once. Don't. Significant behavior changes made quickly, and driven by extreme motivation, are often challenging to implement and maintain. Once that motivation takes a dip, so does one's progress.

Change can be slow and seem minimal at first. But as these new behaviors are practiced over time, healthier experiences are made, and these negative mood states will become less frequent. Therapy with a trained mental health provider can be extremely helpful in targeting and changing unhealthy strategies. They can assist you in becoming more objective to your patterns and habits so that you are able to make necessary changes and adjustments in the moment.

How to
USE THIS BOOK

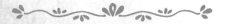

This workbook provides concrete behavior-based exercises, highly applicable to daily life. All strategies are developed from evidence-based therapeutic approaches including Cognitive Behavior Therapy (CBT) and Acceptance and Commitment Therapy (ACT). Research has routinely demonstrated that both are highly successful in changing unhelpful and toxic behaviors.

Exercises are grouped into four chapters, each focusing on a particular stage of pattern and habit change. This book will give you a step-by-step guide on how to identify unhealthy behaviors, modify them, create new habits, and how to maintain them over time. Each exercise is designed to be user-friendly and easily applicable to everyday life, including relationships, family, career, and friendships. Behavior change is a process that has a distinct progression, beginning with the awareness of our behaviors. It is best to follow along in order, as one strategy builds upon the next.

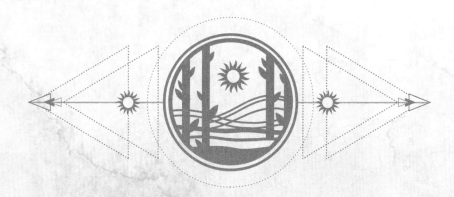

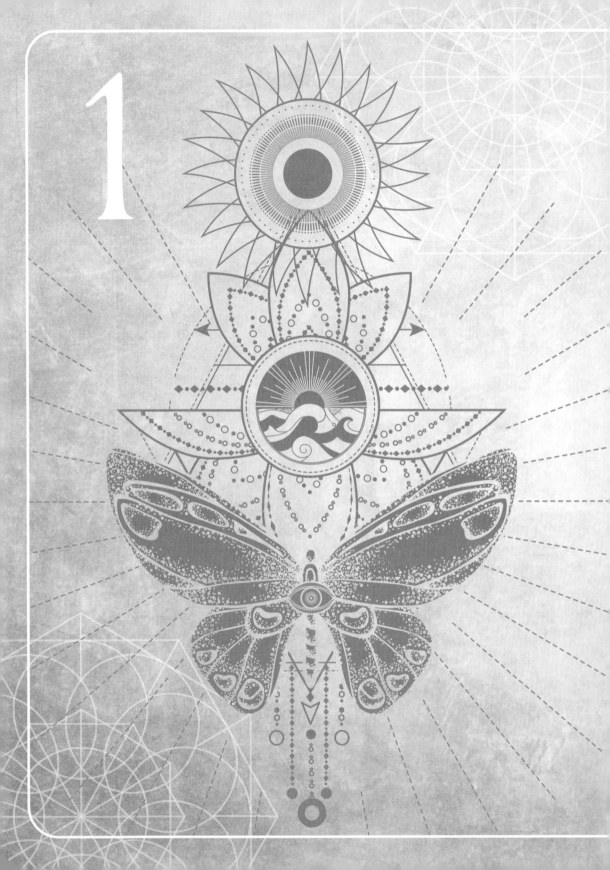

IDENTIFYING YOUR PATTERNS AND HABITS

The first step toward changing patterns and habits is to become aware of them in the first place. When do you do them? What are the triggers? While most habits will have distinct triggers, they are not always within a person's immediate awareness. Because habits are typically automatic in nature, they may seem to just "happen" without any type of cue. But when the behavior loop is slowed down, the triggers become more apparent, giving the person a starting point and sense of control over an aspect of their behavior.

This first chapter will offer strategies on how to slow down your automatic pilot mode, making it easier for you to be aware of your patterns and habits in the moment, identify what types of situations, relationships, and cues trigger the behaviors, and to track their frequency.

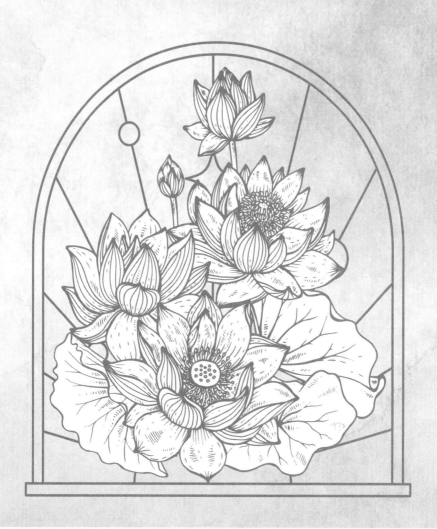

Switching Off
AUTOMATIC PILOT

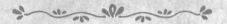

Awareness of one's patterns comes about a little differently. While they don't necessarily have a single identifiable trigger, they do have more relational cues. For example, let's say someone grows up being given the message that nothing they ever do will be good enough. They carry that internalized narrative with them throughout their lives. They may exhibit behaviors such as procrastination and perfectionism, which continue to perpetuate their narrative. The pattern will emerge when a situation or relationship triggers the person's feelings of never being good enough. The current context and longstanding pattern fit together like puzzle pieces.

Awareness of both patterns and habits involves noticing that you are doing the behavior again and switching yourself off automatic pilot. Think about tying your shoes. It is highly likely that you can tie your sneakers while in the middle of a conversation with someone, or while watching something on TV. Because tying your shoes is such a familiar and frequent task, your brain does not need to focus on every step required to make a successful loop. I vividly remember teaching my son how to tie his shoes: such a simple task, yet so difficult to teach. How could this be?

When forced to pay attention to behaviors that have become routine for us, we take ourselves off automatic pilot and become acutely in tune with our actions.

Not only does switching off our automatic pilot mode make us vigilant of our behaviors, but it also makes us highly aware of our emotional states. Habitual behaviors and longstanding patterns don't just require less cognitive awareness, but also less emotional awareness. This is where the concept of "going through the motions" comes from. There is this level of emotional detachment that occurs when we are stuck in a repetitive loop. We check out. Again, this allows our brains to make room for new and unfamiliar stimuli in our environment. But what happens when the entire purpose of our habit or pattern is to *avoid* emotion? What happens to our emotions when we go off automatic pilot? They come flooding in. This is a primary reason why people are so hesitant to change their behaviors. They don't feel equipped to deal with what their patterns and habits have been shielding them from. As you go through this first section, be mindful of emotions that may come up for you. Use it as a source of information about your environment and an indicator that you are very much in the present moment.

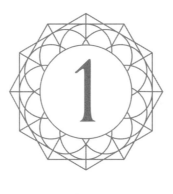

Slow
IT DOWN

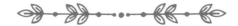

While we may think we recognize all our patterns, many are habitual, and we have little to no awareness of their existence. To become aware of these automatic behaviors, we must slow our brains down and increase our attention in the present moment. Being more present-focused allows us to notice our thoughts, feelings, and behaviors. Pattern change can begin only once we are able to notice these three things objectively in the moment. Once we notice them, we can understand them more effectively and determine which ones are healthy and which ones need modification or elimination. This breathing strategy will teach you how to breathe more effectively, slow your mind down, and become more present-focused.

Proper breathing, known as "belly breathing," allows us to take deeper, more extended breaths from our abdomen rather than breathing from our chest and shoulder area, which results in shorter, shallower breathing. Belly breathing decreases our stress hormones, reminds our bodies that we are safe, and helps us stay in the present moment.

1 Using a mirror or the camera on your phone, position yourself so that you can see your body from the waist up. Stand sideways so that you can see your own profile.

2 Take your normal breath in, and as you do, notice which part of your body moves.

3 Then breathe again, and imagine a blue button resting on top of your belly button. As you breathe in, try to push the blue button off your abdomen. As you exhale, imagine a thread is pulling that blue button back into your abdomen.

4 Practice this breathing strategy for a few minutes twice a day for a week: once in the morning and once in the evening. When first learning this technique, it's best to practice while *not* feeling stressed so that you are able to fully concentrate on proper breathing technique.

5 After each practice, record your experiences. What did you notice? Do you feel different? Is your focus better? Attention improved?

MONDAY

AM:

What did you notice?

Do you feel any changes in your focus or attention?

PM:

What did you notice?

Do you feel any changes in your focus or attention?

TUESDAY

AM:

What did you notice?

Do you feel any changes in your focus or attention?

PM:

What did you notice?

Do you feel any changes in your focus or attention?

WEDNESDAY

AM:

What did you notice?

Do you feel any changes in your focus or attention?

PM:

What did you notice?

Do you feel any changes in your focus or attention?

THURSDAY

AM:

What did you notice?

Do you feel any changes in your focus or attention?

PM:

What did you notice?

Do you feel any changes in your focus or attention?

FRIDAY

AM:

What did you notice?

Do you feel any changes in your focus or attention?

PM:

What did you notice?

Do you feel any changes in your focus or attention?

SATURDAY

AM:

What did you notice?

Do you feel any changes in your focus or attention?

PM:

What did you notice?

Do you feel any changes in your focus or attention?

SUNDAY

AM:

What did you notice?

Do you feel any changes in your focus or attention?

PM:

What did you notice?

Do you feel any changes in your focus or attention?

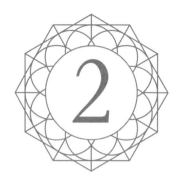

Soak in Your
SURROUNDINGS

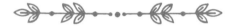

Using your senses to bring your awareness to the present moment
is an extremely effective tool for anchoring yourself.
This exercise is known as the 5-4-3-2-1 strategy.

Using the button breathing skills from page 21,
take a few deep breaths in and out. Then:

5   Notice five things you can see around you.
Say them in your mind or aloud.

4   Notice four things you can touch in your immediate area.
Notice how they feel. Are they soft, rough, slimy?

3   Notice three things you can hear (such as the humming of the
air conditioner).

2   Notice two things you can smell.

1   Notice one thing you can taste. You can do something as simple as
putting your shirt sleeve in your mouth or even tasting your own saliva.

What did you notice while doing this exercise?

....

....

What did you find most difficult about this exercise?

....

....

What are some everyday scenarios where you could benefit from using this strategy?

1. ....

2. ....

3. ....

4. ....

Choose a situation from above to practice this strategy over the next week.
Did you notice any changes to your thoughts and feelings about the situation?
How so?

....

....

As the week progressed, did using this exercise change anything about your
approach to the situation? How?

....

....

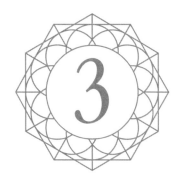

An Apple
FOR THE TEACHER

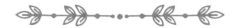

Have you ever been driving home from work, and when you get to your house you have very little recognition of how you actually got there? This is because your brain has gone on automatic pilot mode. When we are engaged in a very familiar, often mundane task like driving a car, we are able to complete it with minimal awareness of our actions. Our brains go offline so that we can attend to other things in our environment. Imagine having to pay attention to every detail of your drive home from work so you don't get lost. This would easily become overwhelming.

There are times, however, when switching off automatic pilot becomes necessary; it's a skill that is essential in recognizing your patterns and habits. This exercise will help you get comfortable with the feeling of turning off your automatic pilot. It will force you to slow down in the moment, making it easier to identify each step involved in a task.

Choose three tasks familiar to you and record them here. In the spaces provided, make a list of all the steps required to complete the task, as if you were teaching it to a class full of students.

Task:

....

Steps to complete:

1. ....
2. ....
3. ....
4. ....
5. ....

Task:

....

Steps to complete:

1. ....
2. ....
3. ....
4. ....
5. ....

Task:

....

Steps to complete:

1. ....
2. ....
3. ....
4. ....
5. ....

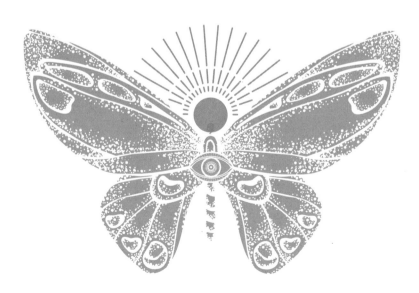

What did you find most difficult about this exercise?

....

....

....

....

....

Did you notice any emotions or thoughts that came up for you (such as frustration)?

....

....

....

....

....

How can this type of awareness of repetitive tasks help you in your day-to-day life?

....

....

....

....

....

Over the next week, choose a different routine for each day and spend a few
minutes practicing with your automatic pilot switch turned off. Pay attention to what
comes up for you while doing the task.

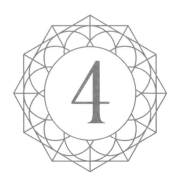

The Opposite
OF INSTINCT

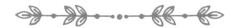

There is way less cognitive and emotional effort required of habits. We go on automatic pilot, which gives our brain more space to take in new information around us. If, however, our habits become detrimental over time, we would need to switch off automatic pilot before any behavior changes can occur. If these changes remain consistent they will eventually become new habits. However, when we experience heightened emotions or stressful times, our brains tend to fall back into what is familiar, which includes old patterns and unhealthy habits. In other words, we switch our automatic pilot back on.

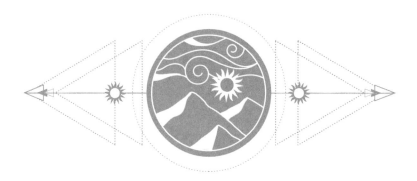

As an example, let's say you broke your right (or dominant) hand during a friendly basketball game. Now, with a cast on your right hand, you are forced to use your left to complete the majority of your daily tasks. The following week, while walking your dog in the park, your dog is suddenly attacked by another dog. In an effort to save your dog, would you grab him back to safety with your left or right hand? Chances are you would instinctively use your right, despite it being broken and in a cast. Why? Because during times of heightened stress, we are more likely to fall back into familiar behavior, even if that's not the healthiest or most effective option. This reversal to automatic pilot conserves cognitive energy so the brain has more available resources to navigate the current stressful situation.

In the spaces provided below, list five basic tasks of daily living (such as brushing your teeth or eating).

1. ....

2. ....

3. ....

4. ....

5. ....

Throughout the day, use your non-dominant hand to complete these tasks. Don't include any tasks that could be dangerous, though, such as driving, riding a bike, working out, and so on.

There are two main goals of this exercise:

1 Becoming mindful of how much cognitive effort you are using to conduct the activities with your non-dominant hand.

2 Noticing when you have gone back to using your dominant hand; specifically, what you were thinking at the time and/or what was occurring around you that left you to go back using your dominant hand.

For each basic task that you listed on the previous page, take a moment to write down what the experience was like to complete the task using your non-dominant hand. How much effort did it take?

1. ....
....

2. ....
....

3. ....
....

4. ....
....

5. ....
....

As best as you can recall, list the thoughts and events that led you to use your dominant hand:

....

....

....

....

Do you notice a particular theme in the above events or thoughts?

....

....

....

Why do you think these specific thoughts and situations put you back on automatic pilot?

....

....

....

....

In the future, how can you use the skills you learned in this exercise to help you notice when you're on automatic pilot?

....

....

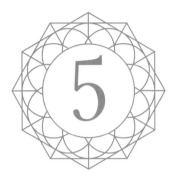

Hello, This Is Your
CAPTAIN SPEAKING

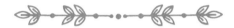

Human beings are notorious for reporting our own behaviors inaccurately, often underestimating or overestimating their frequencies. However, when we shift our awareness to the present moment, we gain a more accurate picture of how often we engage, or don't engage, in a particular behavior.

An important first step in changing patterns and habits is to become aware of how they show up in your daily life. One way to identify these behaviors is to track them. Tracking is an effective way to switch off automatic pilot and bring your awareness directly to what you are doing in the current moment.

The purpose of this exercise is to track when certain habits and patterns occur in your day-to-day. In the spaces provided on the next page, record two personal habits or behavior patterns. Throughout your week, record how often these behaviors occur and write your daily count in the chart on the next page.

Before you begin tracking, provide your best estimate of how often you think these behaviors show up for you during the week.

Pattern/Habit #1:	Pattern/Habit #2:
Estimated # of occurrences per week:	Estimated # of occurrences per week:

PATTERN/ HABIT	SUN	MON	TUE	WED	THU	FRI	SAT
1.							
2.							

How did your estimated number of occurrences compare to the actual count?

....

....

What did you find most difficult about tracking your behaviors over the course of a week?

....

....

Did you notice any patterns in your behaviors as you tracked them?

....

....

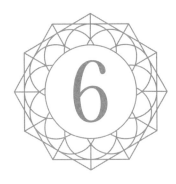

TRACKING TRIGGERS

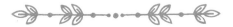

Once your general awareness of your patterns and habits has increased, it becomes important to identify their triggers. These can include places, thoughts, emotions, smells, people, and times of day. Let's use nail-biting as an example. People who bite their nails not only misperceive how frequently they do it, but also when they do it. They are often unaware of what triggers their nail-biting in the moment. Some triggers for nail-biting may include worry, talking to your boss, or taking an exam. Monitoring when habits and patterns are likely to occur allows us to be more proactive about changing them.

Think of two habits you would like to break and record them below.

1. ....

2. ....

List your triggers for each of the two habits.

1. ....   1. ....

2. ....   2. ....

3. ....   3. ....

Choose one set of triggers, and using the chart below, track how often they occur over the course of a week.

TRIGGER	SUN	MON	TUE	WED	THU	FRI	SAT
1.							
2.							
3.							

What did you notice while tracking your triggers?

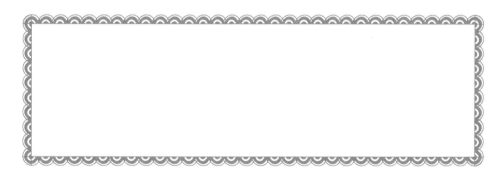

Do you notice any themes within your triggers?

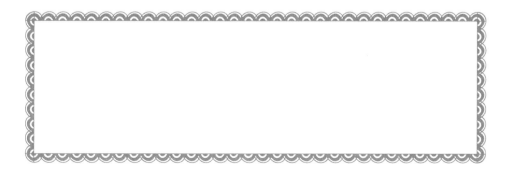

Always
READ THE LABEL

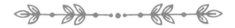

Now that you are more aware of your triggers, it's important to pay attention to the *types* of triggers you are experiencing. Why is this important? Because knowing what kind of trigger you are dealing with ahead of time gives you information on how best to respond. Triggers for habits and other behavior patterns can be emotions, thoughts, anything involving our five senses, places, or people. Take smoking, for example. Common triggers for smoking behavior include stress, other smokers, being out at a bar or restaurant, or even the sensation of hunger.

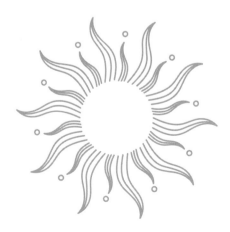

Using all six of the triggers you listed in the previous exercise (see page 36), assign each one to the appropriate label.

☀ Emotions
(e.g., anger):

....

....

☀ Places
(e.g., a bar):

....

....

☀ Thoughts
(e.g., "I sound so stupid"):

....

....

☀ Physical Sensations
(e.g., pain):

....

....

☀ People
(e.g., roommate who also smokes):

....

....

☀ Things
(e.g., a glass of wine):

....

....

Do you notice any themes in your triggers? Do these themes show up in any other areas of your daily life?

....

....

Can you think of any reasons why these themes exist for you or where they may have originated from?

....

....

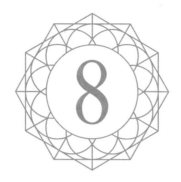

WORDS OF WISDOM

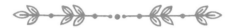

The words we use in our internal dialogue play a key role in how we view ourselves and our abilities. When we are experiencing heightened emotions, we don't always have the cognitive flexibility to devote to abstract grey-area thinking. It's uncertain and requires more effort. Similar to when we fall into familiar patterns of behavior when stressed, the same is true of our thought processes. We tend to engage in all-or-nothing thought called dichotomous thinking. This type of thinking conserves our cognitive energy and allows for quick decision-making under stress. However, when dichotomous thinking is used unnecessarily, it can hinder the process of behavior change and cause us to view ourselves unfavorably (e.g., "I always mess up everything." "I'll never get a promotion no matter what I do.").

Sometimes just changing a word can have a significant impact. For example, consider the use of the words "but" and "and" in a sentence.

"I have to study for my exam *but* it's so hard." vs. "I have to study for my exam *and* it's so hard."

What do you notice?

....

....

The use of the word "but" suggests that the difficulty of the material prevents you from studying. Whereas the use of the word 'and' suggests it is possible for both to occur simultaneously. You can study the material despite it being hard.

Another example is when we utilize words that objectify our thoughts such as "I am…" vs. "I am having the thought…"

"I am a terrible parent." vs. "I'm having the thought that I'm a terrible parent."

What differences do you notice about these two statements?

....

....

The first sentence sounds fact-based: you are a bad parent. The second sentence, however, sounds less "real." By labeling the statement as a thought, it provides objectivity between you and your thinking. You are separate from your thought.

Lastly, some of the words we use suggest that we are unable to perform a particular task because of an emotion. And while our mood can influence our behavior at times, it does not cause them.

"I can't go to my high school reunion because my anxiety is way too bad."

What message does this statement send?

....

....

The sentence suggests that you are unable to go to your reunion because your anxiety is stopping you. While it may feel that way, not going to the reunion is a choice. Yes, you may feel horribly uncomfortable about going, but the anxiety can't physically stop you. If, however, your car broke down, you had a fever, or your childcare fell through, then going to the reunion may not be possible. These are literal obstacles to attending. A feeling, whether anxiety, anger, or sadness, does not literally stop someone from engaging in a behavior.

Think of a specific task or goal that you are currently working towards or plan to in the near future. In the space below, provide a sample sentence for each section with this goal in mind.

But/And:

1. ....

I am/I'm having the thought that:

1. ....

Emotions cause behaviors:

1. ....

Now, provide a corrective response for each example you listed above.

But/And:

1. ....

I am/I'm having the thought that:

1. ....

Emotions cause behaviors:

1. ....

With your goal in mind, do you notice a difference in your perception of yourself and your abilities after revising the statements above?

....

....

Do the revised statements make it more or less likely that you will change your unhealthy habits and patterns? Why?

....

....

Over the next week, try to be mindful of your use of inaccurate self-statements. If you catch yourself, reframe these self-statements in a healthier way and notice if it changes your perceptions and/or behaviors in the moment. In the tracking chart below, record any negative statements you make, along with your healthy, reframed statement. Also, provide a brief description of your surroundings at the time (e.g., who are you with, what are you doing). This can help you become more proactive in identifying unproductive statements.

MONDAY	
TUESDAY	
WEDNESDAY	
THURSDAY	
FRIDAY	
SATURDAY	
SUNDAY	

Interpersonal INVENTORY

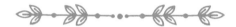

Just as habits are present in our daily routines, patterns of behavior can be found in our relationships. This includes family, friends, coworkers, and significant others. While some of our patterns are beneficial, others may keep us locked in toxic cycles. Some relational patterns that worked quite well for us while growing up within our family may not be effective in our adult lives. As the circumstances of our lives change, our behaviors must shift and adjust accordingly. Without ongoing evaluation of the patterns in our daily lives, we run the risk of getting stuck in the repetitiveness of unhealthy dynamics.

An effective way to increase awareness of our relationship patterns is to map them out. Something I like to use often with my patients is what I call an "Interpersonal Inventory (II)." An II is exactly what it sounds like: it is an inventory of your relationships across all areas of your life. It allows you to identify the people with whom you have relationships, but also enables you to examine the underlying patterns of each dynamic.

In the spaces provided on the next page, list the names of all the people with whom you have relatively close relationships.

WORK	FAMILY

FRIENDS	DATING

Take a minute to think about your relationships with the people you've identified above. For each relationship, answer the following six questions on the next two pages. (If you run out of space, you can answer these questions in your personal journal.)

WORK

1 How long has this relationship existed?

2 Has this relationship shifted over time? If so, how?

3 How would you describe the relationship? Is it toxic? Healthy? Rewarding?

4 If you could change anything about this relationship, what would it be?

5 Is this change something that they would need to make, or you?

6 Does this relationship offer you something beneficial? Does it take *away* something bad?

FAMILY

1 How long has this relationship existed?

2 Has this relationship shifted over time? If so, how?

3 How would you describe the relationship? Is it toxic? Healthy? Rewarding?

4 If you could change anything about this relationship, what would it be?

5 Is this change something that they would need to make, or you?

6 Does this relationship offer you something beneficial? Does it take *away* something bad?

FRIENDS

1 How long has this relationship existed?

2 Has this relationship shifted over time? If so, how?

3 How would you describe the relationship? Is it toxic? Healthy? Rewarding?

4 If you could change anything about this relationship, what would it be?

5 Is this change something that they would need to make, or you?

6 Does this relationship offer you something beneficial? Does it take *away* something bad?

DATING

1 How long has this relationship existed?

2 Has this relationship shifted over time? If so, how?

3 How would you describe the relationship? Is it toxic? Healthy? Rewarding?

4 If you could change anything about this relationship, what would it be?

5 Is this change something that they would need to make, or you?

6 Does this relationship offer you something beneficial? Does it take *away* something bad?

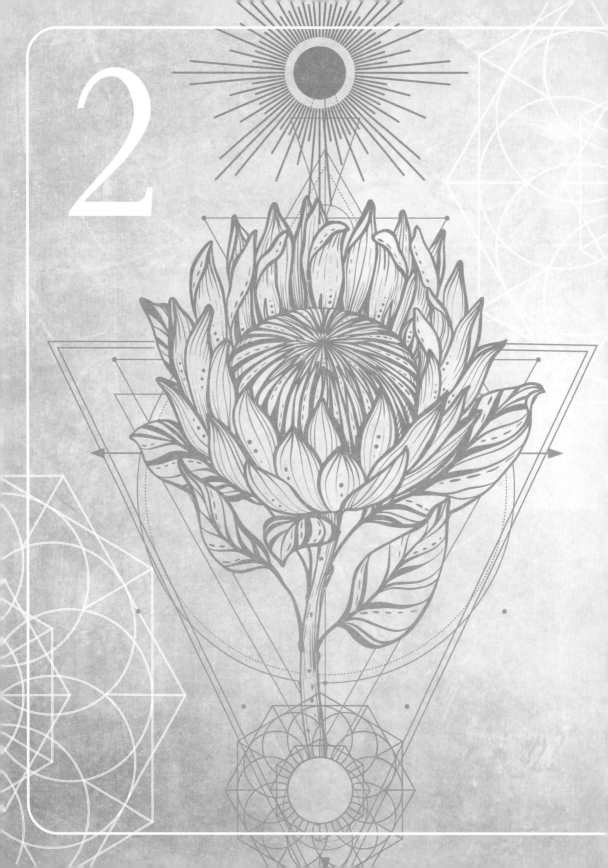

HEALTHY
OR HURTFUL?

We all have patterns and habits, many of which developed during childhood in response to the world around us. Growing up, we model that which is familiar to us, that which usually comes from our parents and caregivers. There are numerous benefits to establishing patterned behavior and habits. Think of patterns and habits as brain energy savers. They allow our brains to focus on other things that may be more difficult, new, or exciting. They also offer a sense of structure and routine. We gravitate toward familiarity and feel more in control when we can predict what comes next in any given moment. Take your morning routine, for example. You know what to expect from the period when you wake up until you leave your house. Over time, this routine becomes habitual; you don't have to put forth much cognitive effort to determine what comes next, like washing your face or getting dressed. Having this routine also allows you to attend to other things that may need your attention—such as a company presentation, a final exam, or an unexpected emergency.

This chapter will help you identify which of your patterns and habits are healthy, and which are not. These exercises will give you a better understanding of why you engage in certain behaviors and the reasons why you continue to maintain unhealthy habits and patterns.

Keep
OR LET GO

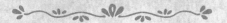

When patterns or habits are no longer making your life easier, it becomes necessary to modify, change, or get rid of those behaviors. In other words, they need to be flexible over time as our lives and environments change. What once was effective for you growing up may no longer work for you in adulthood. Formerly healthy behaviors may now appear unhealthy in your current environment. This can leave a person feeling stuck or anxious, and even place them at risk for depression and substance abuse. It can also lead to toxic relationships with others.

Obviously, not all patterns and habits become unhealthy over time, nor do they require adjustment. Some behaviors retain their healthy function across a lifespan. It's likely that you are already engaging in several healthy habits and behavior patterns. Healthy eating, staying hydrated daily, and maintaining a clean work and home environment all represent healthy habits.

Just like many habit-forming behaviors, not all patterns are unhealthy,

either. Let's look at the way someone might manage uncomfortable emotions at work, such as stress and anxiety. Maybe they take some time to gather their thoughts or go on a walk to cool down before sending an email to their boss, perhaps they closely monitor their tone of voice and make sure their body language is non-threatening, and they suggest a meeting so all parties can openly discuss their concerns. This would be considered an extremely healthy pattern of behavior.

Understanding which behaviors are enhancing your life versus those that are limiting is critical in improving mood, productivity, and relationships. Oftentimes, the behaviors that are most unhealthy are the ones most familiar to you (such as people pleasing), while the most comforting behaviors can sometimes be the most toxic (such as smoking). Understanding this concept allows you to be more objective to your own behaviors and gives you the space to make changes and monitor your progress over time.

Revisiting
YOUR VALUES

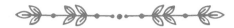

One of the most important steps in changing behavior patterns and habits is to take a step back and reassess your values. Do your behaviors reflect your values? Or do your actions take you in the opposite direction? Do you even know what your values are?

It is also important to differentiate between your goals and your values. Goals are action-based end points. They are tangible and achievable markers. For example, a goal might be to run a marathon, or to run a marathon and finish in the top ten. Values are more abstract (such as prioritizing an active and healthy lifestyle). Values dictate the types of goals you set. In other words, if you train to run your first marathon, you are doing something that takes you closer to your value of living an active and healthy life.

This exercise will help you differentiate between goals and values and examine if your behaviors are consistent with your values.

In the spaces below, list four things that you value most in life. Try to be as specific as possible. For example, instead of saying, "I value being a good parent," you can say, "I value being a present and attentive parent to my children."

1. ....

2. ....

3. ....

4. ....

For each value listed above, provide a real-life example of one behavior that is in line with your value and one behavior that goes against it. For example, reading to your children at bedtime is a behavior that could be consistent with being a present parent. Scrolling through Instagram while putting your child to bed may be a behavior that is inconsistent with your value.

1. a. ....

   b. ....

2. a. ....

   b ....

3. a. ....

   b. ....

4. a. ....

   b. ....

Write down three goals that take you closer to one of the values you listed above.

1. ....

2. ....

3. ....

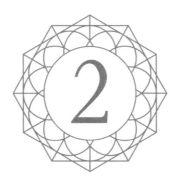

The Habit OF GRATITUDE

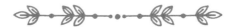

Gratitude has been shown to not only have a positive impact on how we think and feel, but also on our behaviors. Acknowledging what you are grateful for can lead to higher levels of confidence, motivation, and optimism, making behavior change more likely to occur, and be maintained, in your day-to-day. Even simple, daily acknowledgments of appreciation can motivate behavior change and help you achieve your goal. There are several ways in which gratitude can be expressed. Some examples include listing three things you are grateful for every day, keeping a gratitude journal, taking a few minutes each day to be mindfully present while appreciating everything in the moment, showing appreciation to a friend by buying them coffee, or simply making a conscious effort to say thank you.

Every day for the next week, commit to showing gratitude to yourself or to someone else. You may use any of the examples listed above or come up with your own. You can use the same expression of gratitude daily or implement a variety of strategies. Remember, the key is to be consistent. Who knows? Maybe you will end up making gratitude a daily habit.

List five ways in which you can express gratitude towards yourself:

1. ....
2. ....
3. ....
4. ....
5. ....

List five ways in which you can express gratitude to others:

1. ....
2. ....
3. ....
4. ....
5. ....

	SUN	MON	TUE	WED	THU	FRI	SAT
Expressions of gratitude used.							
Observations during act of gratitude. What did you notice while expressing gratitude?							
Observations post-act of gratitude. What did you notice after expressing gratitude?							

At the end of the week, record your responses to the following questions.

As you practiced gratitude throughout the week, what common themes did you notice in your thinking and mood?

....

....

....

Did you find that gratitude became easier to express as your week progressed? Why or why not?

....

....

....

Did you notice any healthy changes in your daily behaviors that could be attributed to expressing gratitude? Or maybe an existing healthy habit that became easier to maintain?

....

....

....

If you weren't already doing so, how likely are you now to implement gratitude into your daily routine? How do you see it benefiting you?

....

....

....

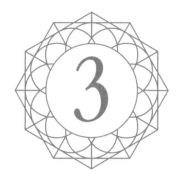

Focus on
FUNCTION FIRST

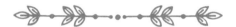

Every pattern and habit has a function, which is the underlying reason behind why we do what we do. Simply put, the reason we engage in a pattern, habit, or behavior is because it gives us something good. If it didn't, we wouldn't continue to repeat it. For example, say you have made it a habit to turn your phone off every evening an hour before bed to improve sleep. Because this habit has improved your sleep, you are more likely to repeat it. In other words, this habit gave you something good: better sleep.

How, then, would this apply to unhealthy habits and behaviors that don't seem to give us anything good in return? Take, for example, food addiction. This habit is unhealthy and can have serious emotional and physical consequences. So why is it difficult to change? Because it *does* give something good in return: food addiction temporarily takes away one's emotional pain. It offers a rush and a false sense of control and safety in the moment. It's this temporary emotional avoidance, this distraction from pain, that is the underlying function of most unhealthy behavior patterns and habits.

These exercises will help you identify the underlying function of your behaviors
and gain a better understanding of how to differentiate between those
that are healthy and unhealthy.

In the space below, provide examples of your unhealthy habits and patterns.

1. ....

2. ....

3. ....

4. ....

For each of the above behaviors, ask yourself the following question: "What is this
particular behavior giving me that's good?"

1. ....

2. ....

3. ....

4. ....

Take a minute to review your responses. Do you notice a theme?

....

....

....

....

....

....

....

....

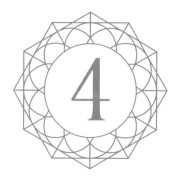

HIGHWAY DRIVING

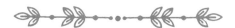

Giving up patterns or habits can be scary. The thought of changing behaviors, even when toxic, can be a daunting task. Most people are unaware that it can be their own behavior patterns causing them distress. We often will engage in habits and patterns that help us to avoid the things we don't want to think or feel. The behaviors that routinely help us to avoid internal discomfort are more often than not going to be unhelpful and possibly toxic (for example, drinking alcohol when sad, excessive worry when we feel out of control). The more we try to get rid of uncomfortable thoughts and feelings, the longer they stick around and the heavier they feel. Even though it's uncomfortable, it is best to remain present-focused and look *at* your thoughts rather than battle against them. This is known as cognitive defusion. It is a strategy that helps us look at our thoughts and feelings as if we were seeing them on a billboard while driving along a highway. Instead of being entangled with your internal dialogue, you place it outside of you, allowing you to look *at* it rather than be consumed by it. This allows our discomfort to pass sooner and easier, and helps us engage in healthy behaviors that align with our values rather than ones that serve an avoidant function.

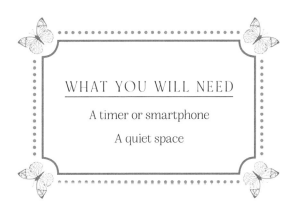

WHAT YOU WILL NEED

A timer or smartphone

A quiet space

For sixty seconds, just sit and be present. Focus on your surroundings and use your breathing to ground you in the moment. As thoughts come into your head, rather than pushing them away, using distraction, or engaging with them, simply notice them and let them pass.

As you do this, picture yourself driving along a highway. All along the side of the road are billboards. When thoughts come into your mind, look at them as if they are written on these. You wouldn't stop your car suddenly at each billboard to read it, nor would you try to get rid of the billboard. You would continue driving along in your car, noticing them as you passed by. The same approach should be taken with our thinking. By looking at your thoughts, rather than being tangled up with them, you can be more present-focused and aware of your environment, including your own behaviors.

Make a list below of three habits you would like to break.

1. ....

2. ....

3. ....

Using the billboard strategy, notice how frequently you engage in these behaviors and record it in the weekly chart. Pay attention to how the defusion technique impacted your ability to observe your own behaviors in the moment.

	SUN	MON	TUE	WED	THU	FRI	SAT
Habit 1:							
Habit 2:							
Habit 3:							

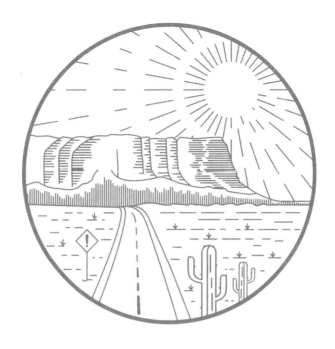

What did you notice during this exercise? What feelings and thoughts came up for you?

....

....

....

Was the defusion technique helpful when being objective to your thoughts? Why?

....

....

....

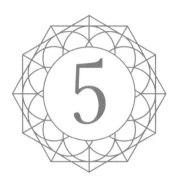

No Longer
IN SERVICE

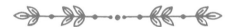

Patterns and habits are typically longstanding behaviors stemming from childhood. They guide and influence how we interact with others, our environment, and even ourselves. Some patterns continue to benefit us into adulthood, while others do not. Unhelpful patterns, while at one time healthy, now become ineffective, leading to relationship difficulties, anxiety, stress, and depression.

When changing behavioral patterns, it is beneficial to look at their origins: the how and why they developed. And while knowing where our patterns stem from isn't necessary for behavior change, it helps to know that at one point, this pattern *did* work, it made sense and was healthy. It provides a context to understand why we do what we do.

Think about a habit or pattern you really would like to change but are scared to let go of, then record it below.

....

In what situation do you find yourself routinely engaging in this pattern?

....

If you did not engage in this pattern/habit in the scenario you listed above, what are you *fearful* may happen? How likely is this to occur?

....

....

If it was 100% guaranteed that your fear would never happen, would you be more willing to change your pattern or habit? Why?

....

....

Can you think of another time(s) in your life when you felt this same fear? Describe it.

....

....

Do you notice any themes or similarities?

....

....

Would your current pattern make sense in your most feared situation? Why?

....

....

Even when our patterns are no longer useful to us, we tend to hold on to them. We are comfortable with their familiarity, and they feel safe. And why wouldn't they? They did work at one point. We continue to use unnecessary patterns because we think the current situation has the same context as the one our pattern originated from. It doesn't. Yet we respond to it as if it does.

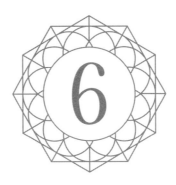

Putting Values
TO WORK

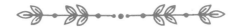

Now that you have a more in-depth understanding of your values, let's put it into practice. A core component of both habit and behavior change is being able to recognize, in the moment, when your behaviors take you away from your values. When emotionally heightened, it can be difficult to pause and redirect your actions. When we are stressed, tired, or angry, our brains are at maximum capacity, leaving very little room to assess the quality of our behaviors. This exercise will help you notice when your behaviors and values are not in-sync and teach you to make more value-driven choices.

Over the next week, pay close attention to when you engage in behaviors that take you away from your values. What is going on around you? Who are you with? What are you thinking/feeling?

Record your observations below and on the next page whenever you catch yourself engaging in behaviors that are opposite to your values.

Identify the avoidant behaviors:

1. ....

2. ....

Details of the current situation:

1. ....

2. ....

Did these behaviors initially make you feel better?

....

Did they take away any negative emotions or get rid of negative thoughts? If so, what were they?

....

Are these common behavior patterns for you?   ◯ Yes   ◯ No

What would be alternative, healthier, value-based behaviors?

1. ....

2. ....

3. ....

4. ....

Would any of these alternative behaviors have changed the situation and/or affected the outcome? How so?

1. ....

2. ....

3. ....

4. ....

Relationship ROADMAP

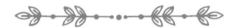

When changing our patterns and habits, it is essential to examine our interpersonal patterns. Think of each relationship as a dance, with each person having a particular role. When one partner steps right, the other goes left; one goes up, the other goes down. It's habitual and predictable. This dance is the pattern. When we can understand the *dance,* we are better able to identify what needs to be changed in hopes of making the relationship healthier. It is important to consider our perception of the relationship's quality. This alerts us as to whether a relational pattern is healthy. It is also important to keep in mind, however, that sometimes patterns we perceive as "good" may just be familiar and comfortable, not necessarily healthy.

Using your examples from the Interpersonal Inventory exercise (see page 44), choose eight of the relationships you listed. On the bidirectional arrows that connect you to each of the outside circles, label the relationship as either + (healthy), – (toxic), or = (neutral).

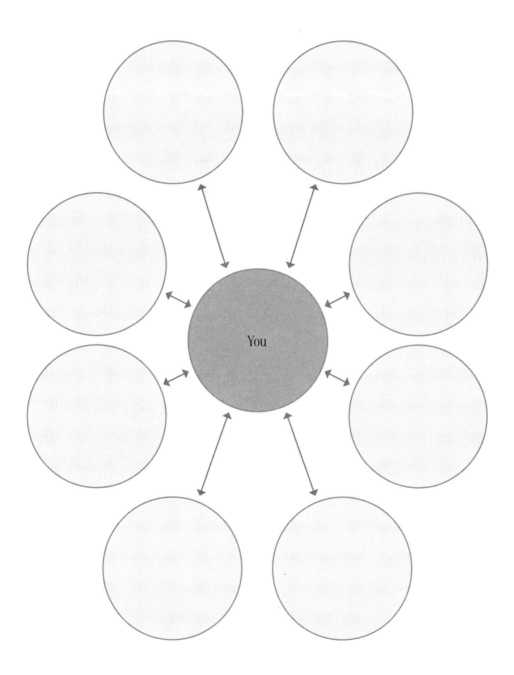

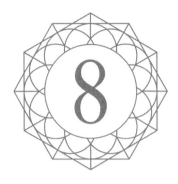

Dance Like Everyone
IS WATCHING

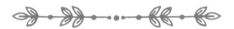

In this exercise, you'll continue the analysis of your relationships that you began in the previous exercise (see page 68). Pick any three of the relationships you labeled as toxic (–) and provide an example of an interpersonal pattern you share with that individual. For example, let's say that whenever you do something for yourself (such as go on vacation, say no to doing a favor) you are called selfish or obnoxious by this person. Or instead of repeatedly telling your teenager to clean their room, you just clean it for them because you don't want to argue.

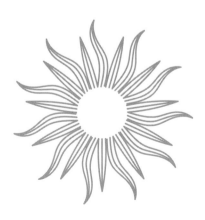

1. ....
   ....
   ....
   ....

2. ....
   ....
   ....
   ....

3. ....
   ....
   ....
   ....

What was your experience teasing out your relationship patterns?
Did you find it difficult?

....

....

Did any of the pattern dynamics you noticed surprise you?

....

....

Are there any similarities and/or differences you observed across your relationships?
Did you notice any emerging themes?

....

....

Familiarity is Not Always YOUR FRIEND

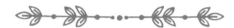

Patterns of behavior are often the longstanding routines with people in our lives. Why, though, do we continue to engage in these patterns with others if it is unhealthy for us? Familiarity. It is comfortable, predictable, and feels easier. But while it may feel easier in the moment, it is only helping us avoid the discomfort of change. This continues to foster unhealthy behaviors, uncomfortable emotions, and toxic relationships.

For each of the examples you listed in the previous exercise (see page 70), think about what it is that you are avoiding by continuing with the pattern (such as feelings, responses of others, thoughts). For example, when you clean your kid's room rather than asking them to because you don't want to argue, what are you *really* avoiding by doing it yourself?

1. ....

   ....

2. ....

   ....

3. ....

....

For each of the answers you gave above, think about an alternative response that wouldn't allow you to avoid any internal discomfort. In the previous example, let's say you tell your teen to clean her room. She replies no, yelling at you that you are annoying and she "hates you." Yes, you may feel guilt; you may feel an overwhelming urge to clean her room to avoid how you feel. Instead, however, you sit with these feelings *and* at the same go out to run an errand rather than clean the room. In the spaces below, record an alternative response pattern to each of your situations.

1. ....

....

2. ....

....

3. ....

....

Throughout the week, test out your alternative responses. Pay attention to what comes up for you. Is it uncomfortable? Scary? Unfamiliar?

....

How does the other person in the dynamic respond? Do they respond appropriately? Do they get defensive? Angry? Or do they increase the intensity of their typical response?

....

Identifying what you are avoiding is a critical first step in changing your relational patterns. Developing alternative responses that force you to sit with your discomfort leads to much healthier relationships. The more willing you are to tolerate these feelings, the more effective you will be in breaking unhealthy relational habits.

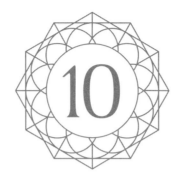

OUT OF TIME

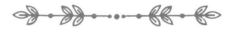

Not only do unhealthy habits and patterns take us away from our values and lead to increased stress, but they use a considerable amount of mental energy and effort, too. Most unhealthy behaviors also result in negative consequences. Navigating these outcomes can become all-consuming, taking us away, yet again, from our values, and creating a vicious cycle. Unhealthy habits and patterns can be emotionally, mentally, and even physically taxing. They take us out of the present moment and away from the things we enjoy and value.

This exercise will give you a greater awareness of how much of your time is consumed by unhealthy patterns and habits and help you identify more adaptive behaviors.

In the spaces below, write down a few examples of unhealthy habits or patterns you have.

1. ....

2. ....

3. ....

4. ....

Over the next week, pay attention to how often these habits and patterns arise in your day-to-day. Record the frequency in the chart below. In addition, at the end of each day, record the total time you spent immersed in these unhealthy patterns or habits.

Habit/Pattern	SUN	MON	TUE	WED	THU	FRI	SAT
1.							
2.							
3.							
4.							
Actual time spent							

What was your experience while tracking these behaviors? What did you notice?

....

....

Add up the total amount of time you spent engaged in these behaviors over the entire week. What comes up for you if you were told to immediately abandon them?

....

....

If you had the opportunity to get back the time you spent engaging in your unhealthy habits and patterns, what would you choose to do instead? What would you do more of? Less of?

....

....

....

Do you notice any themes in your tracking chart? Is there a particular day you spent more time engaged in your pattern? Maybe a specific time during the week?

....

....

....

Think about what was occurring at these heightened times. Was something upsetting you? Were you stressed? Who was around you in that moment?

....

....

Now that you are more aware of how often you engage in these unhealthy patterns and habits, choose two and track them again over another week.

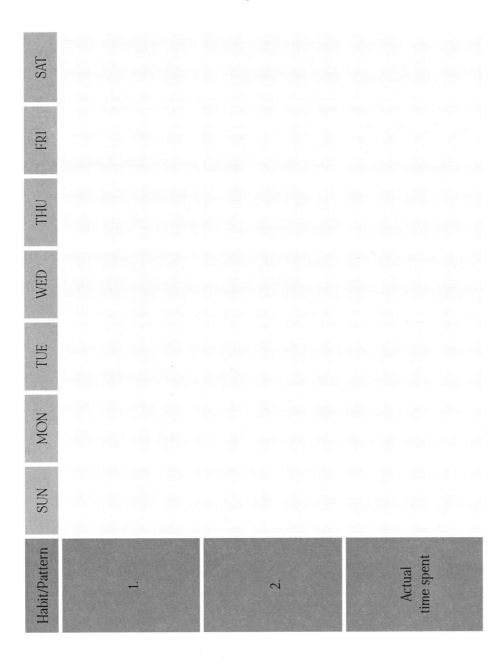

Habit/Pattern	SUN	MON	TUE	WED	THU	FRI	SAT
1.							
2.							
Actual time spent							

Did you engage in these behaviors less? What did you choose to do instead?

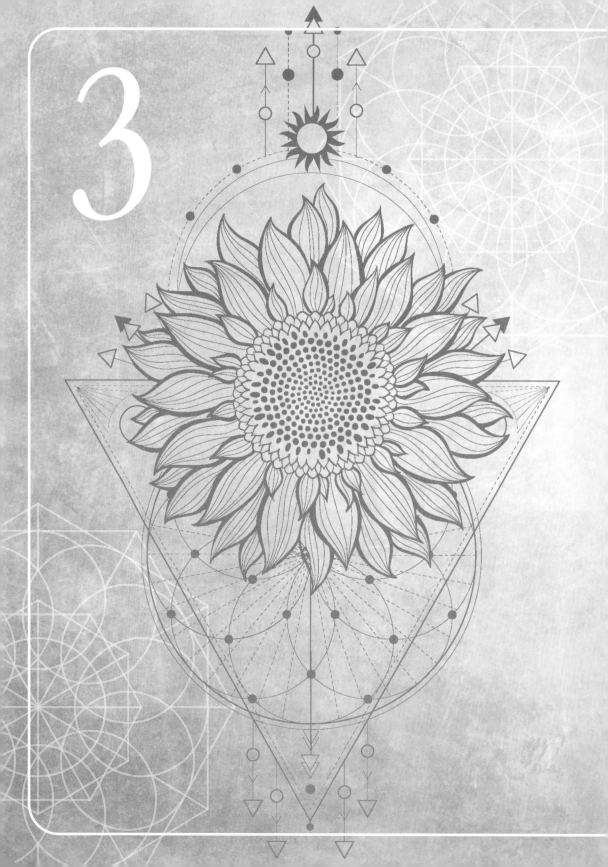

CHANGING UNHEALTHY HABITS AND PATTERNS

Changing unhealthy habits and patterns can be extremely difficult, especially when they have been in place for a long time. It's for this reason that we often gravitate toward familiar behaviors; they feel safe and predictable. Behavior change is further complicated by people shying away from change. We are creatures of habit. Change, even if for the better, can be scary and cause feelings of uncertainty. If I change a longstanding behavior, will I fall apart? How will I put myself back together? This is why so many people are resistant to change. It is exceedingly difficult to give up the familiar, yet unhealthy, comfort that your habits and patterns provided.

This chapter will teach you how to establish achievable and measurable goals in your effort to change habits and patterns. It will also give you helpful strategies to engage in meaningful change and eventually establish healthier habits and patterns.

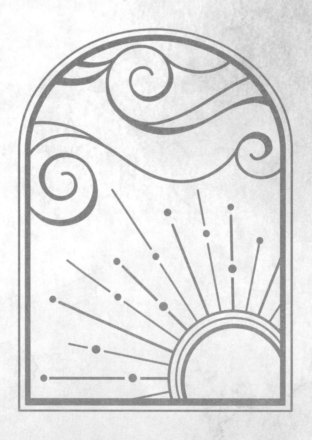

Set Measurable Goals
FOR CHANGE

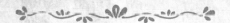

When attempting to change or alter your habits and patterns, it is critical to first establish goals. Trying to change behaviors without establishing achievable and measurable goals creates a level of uncertainty and anxiety that can set us up for failure. Similarly, trying to tackle too much change at once can feel overwhelming and scary. Taking on a new task in small stages makes it less likely that a person will quit or resort to old patterns. Forming new patterns and habits, in small steps, creates a sense of mastery and accomplishment. The reinforcement of this new behavior is what makes it more likely to happen again. When we try to change or take on too much at once, we sometimes "white knuckle" through it, meaning we push through it begrudgingly, never really being in the moment. Our sense of mastery is minimized, and so it is less likely we will repeat the new behavior.

When initiating any type of habit or pattern change, be mindful of the role others play in your life. For example, let's say you are in the process of getting sober after fifteen years of alcohol abuse. For those fifteen years, you played a particular role within your family and social circles. Addiction has a systemic influence, meaning your addiction impacts the lives of everyone around you. People may have isolated themselves from you, you may have isolated yourself from others, some people may have been enablers. In other words, everyone played a specific part within your social dynamic.

When one person makes changes within a system, it throws the entire dynamic off-kilter. Typically, this results in a form of pushback from others. When actively changing your behaviors, you may hear things like "You seem different," "You're being selfish," or "Why are you so angry?" The function of these statements is to attempt to push you back into your original role. Why? Because that's how everyone else feels most comfortable.

Goals:
A TRILOGY

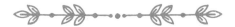

When changing behavior, specifying our goals gives us a game plan for how best to reach our destination point. Goals help us with two main things when breaking habits or forming new patterns. First, they keep us on track. Second, they provide us with a sense of accomplishment, mastery, and confidence in our ability to change our behaviors.

Goals can be broken down into three types: immediate, short-term, and long-term. Immediate goals are anything you can do right now to either prepare you or put you on track to achieve a short-term goal. A short-term goal is, in a sense, a small part of your long-term goal. Think of it as a rest stop along a highway. To get to wherever it is you are going, you must fill up your tank along the way. Without this fuel, you won't make it to your destination (or at least not easily). It is often the accumulation of short-term goals that leads to a long-term goal achievement. Long-term goals are those that are in line with your values; when achieved, they enhance your life. Long-term goals typically reflect a milestone, something you have been working on for an extended period that has been a focal point in your life.

Think about a long-term goal you have been working toward or wish to achieve, then record it below.

....

....

....

Now, write down three examples of short-term goals that are associated with your long-term goal.

1. ....

2. ....

3. ....

For each of the short-term goals above, give an example of one immediate goal that you could begin to work on now.

1. ....

2. ....

3. ....

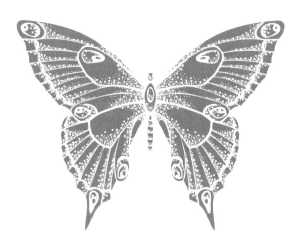

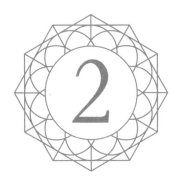

Prioritize
YOUR PLAN

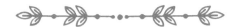

The journey of breaking habits and changing toxic patterns can be an exciting one, but it can also be daunting. Uncomfortable emotions may emerge, and doubts appear that could impact your willingness to continue. An excellent way to limit the occurrence of intense negative thoughts and feelings is to prioritize your goals. Not everything is equally important, timely, or necessary. This exercise will teach you how to prioritize your goals so that you do not become overwhelmed.

Think about all the things on your plate at this moment that you need to deal with. These do not have to be related to changing or modifying habits or patterns. They can simply be going to the grocery store or meeting a work project deadline next week. In the space provided, list eight items that require your attention.

1. ....
2. ....
3. ....
4. ....

5. ....

6. ....

7. ....

8. ....

Next to each item, give it a rating of one to eight; one being the least pressing to eight being the most. Each item must get a number and you may not use a number more than once.

What was your experience as you rated your tasks?

....

....

....

Throughout your week, keep a record of the tasks and responsibilities that come up for you. Give each a number, with one being the least pressing. It is important to be flexible when prioritizing tasks, since our days and schedules shift so frequently. As additional things are added to your plate and others are taken off, make sure to routinely assess and prioritize your to-do list. This will prevent you from becoming easily overwhelmed, and give you structure and a sense of control over your day-to-day life.

Does prioritizing your goals and tasks make the process of accomplishing them less overwhelming? Do you notice a difference in your mood and productivity compared to prior efforts?

....

....

....

....

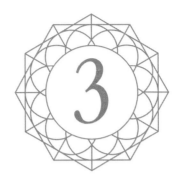

Moods
ARE NOT GOALS

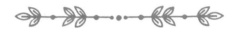

Whenever I work with my patients on defining their goals, I always use the example of "being happy." It makes sense. People come to therapy to be happier in their lives. But what exactly *is* happiness? Happiness is an abstract concept, and abstract concepts make bad goals. "Calm" is not a good goal. "Healthier" is not a good goal. Abstract goals are nothing more than moving targets, and ones that you will never consistently meet. Here's why.

First, mood states are fluid. It is not possible to experience one mood all the time. Mood states themselves are not bad. They are not dangerous. While they may influence our behaviors, they don't actually *stop* us from doing them. You are able to feel anxious and at the same time go to work.

Second, mood-based, abstract goals mean different things at different times to different people. For example, let's say your goal is to change your unhealthy lifestyle and create healthier habits. If this were *my* goal, it might include playing tennis, cooking more, and walking. But for you, this may mean watching fewer TikTok videos, spending less time watching TV, and drinking less alcohol. Setting a goal of "being healthier" without clearly defining what that means for *you* can set you up for unrealistic expectations and the risk of not achieving your goals.

We need to "operationally define" our goals, meaning we need to clearly define what, how, when, and how often. Think of "healthy" as an umbrella, and your goals as all the things that would go under this umbrella. Goals should always be achievable, measurable, and definitive.

HEALTHY

Healthy:

1 Cook two healthy meals two times a week. Did I do it?   ◯ Yes ◯ No

2 Walk for ten minutes two times a week. Did I do it?   ◯ Yes ◯ No

3 Turn off my phone at 8 pm three times a week. Did I do it?   ◯ Yes ◯ No

If someone else were to look at your goals, are they objective and replicable? Are all these goals specific, measurable, and easier to achieve than "I want to be healthy"?

Think of a goal you wish to work toward and record it below. This can be a habit you wish to break, a toxic pattern you want to adjust, or anything else you want to change.

Goal: ....

List four defined goals that fall under your umbrella goal:

1. ....

2. ....

3. ....

4. ....

Does each goal above allow for a yes/no outcome? If not, how can you revise them so that they do?

....

....

If you shared these goals with someone else, are they objective and replicable? If not, how can you revise them so that they are?

....

....

Now that you have clearly articulated goals, let's put them into practice. Choose an umbrella goal that you want to work toward. You can use your goal listed above or pick a different one. Under your umbrella, list four definitive and replicable sub-goals. Choose one of the four to focus on for a week and track your progress in the chart on the next page. At the end of each day you'll tally up your behaviors so that you have a tangible outcome. At the end of the week, note how much time you spent in total.

Did you achieve your goal? ◯ Yes ◯ No

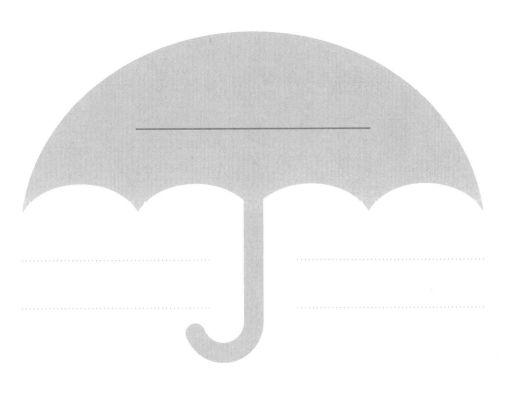

Day of the week	Time spent working towards sub-goal	Actual time spent
SUN		
MON		
TUE		
WED		
THU		
FRI		
SAT		

No Shaming
IN MAINTAINING

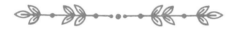

When changing habits and patterns, we tend to set the difficulty level of our goals prematurely and/or unrealistically. Sometimes maintaining your current progress is just as effective and meaningful as setting a brand-new behavioral goal. For example, let's say you have been working towards the goal to live a healthier lifestyle with healthier habits, and part of that umbrella goal is to go to the gym three times per week. For the last two months, you have been doing that successfully. You may now want to increase it to four times per week, which is reasonable if your life allows for that. In other words, what if you don't have childcare on that fourth day, or what if you can't afford to take an additional workout class? It is important to take current life circumstances into account when revising or setting behavioral goals. Instead of going four times a week and potentially setting yourself up for failure, set your goal to *maintain* where you are currently at: keep going to the gym three times a week. This continues to boost confidence and mastery and reduces potential feelings of defeat.

Think of some goals you are currently working toward, or plan to soon, and record them below.

1. ....
2. ....
3. ....

For each of the goals above, what would be the next level?

1. ....
2. ....
3. ....

Which of the revised goals above do you think might prove to be unrealistic for you at this point in time?

....

Why so? (for example, time restrictions, finances, interest)

....

If you try to move to the next level anyway, what do you anticipate may happen?

....
....

If your prediction turned out to be correct, would this make it more or less likely that you would continue trying to achieve this goal? Why?

....
....

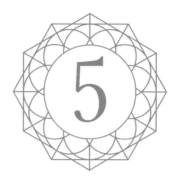

Meaningful MODIFICATION

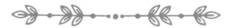

When changing a habit or behavior, people often choose a brand-new goal, something that is either absent from their lives or that is drastically different. This can be fine within reason, but sometimes these goals are too much to tackle at once and can lead to you becoming discouraged and giving up. What if, instead of setting a brand-new behavior as a goal, you modify an existing behavior? For example, using the umbrella goal of being "healthier," let's say you set a very realistic and objective goal of going to the gym two times a week. But you hate the gym. In fact, you haven't set foot in a gym for twenty years. Why put yourself at risk for failure when you can obtain the same feeling of accomplishment by setting a goal that is a variation of an existing healthy behavior? For example, you already take a yoga class once a week that you thoroughly enjoy. So why not add in a different type of yoga to your routine? You are still achieving your goal of becoming healthier, and you're doing something in line with your values that fulfills you. And the more consistent you are, the higher the likelihood of it becoming a habit.

In the spaces provided, record a potential variation for each existing goal.

For example:

Umbrella goal: To live a healthier lifestyle.
Existing behavioral goal: I cook three healthy meals per week.
Variation: Continue to cook three healthy meals per week, but try different recipes.

Umbrella goal: Become more fiscally responsible.

Existing behavioral goal: I set aside $50 per week into my savings account.

Variation:..

Umbrella goal: Be more social with my friends.

Existing behavioral goal: I attend book club once per week.

Variation:..

Umbrella goal: Become more present in my relationships.

Existing behavioral goal: I leave my phone off while out to dinner.

Variation:..

Record three of your own umbrella and existing goals below. Come up with a variation goal for each that increases the likelihood you would achieve your goals.

Umbrella goal: ....

Existing goal: ....

Variation: ....

Umbrella goal: ....

Existing goal: ....

Variation: ....

Umbrella goal: ....

Existing goal: ....

Variation: ....

In looking at these new variations, what do you anticipate would happen to your motivation to continue working toward your goal? Does it increase? Decrease? Have no impact?

....

....

....

Let's test out if your variation goals benefit your progress. Using the chart below, record how frequently you engage in a variation of an existing goal.

Habit/Pattern	SUN	MON	TUE	WED	THU	FRI	SAT
1.							
2.							
3.							
Actual time spent							

After completing your tracking for the week, note how much time you spent in total and answer the following items:

What did you notice while tracking your behaviors? What thoughts and feelings came up for you?

....

....

....

Do variations change how you view your ability to achieve your overarching goals? How so?

....

....

....

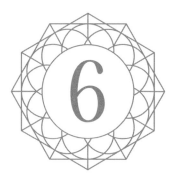

PUT IT ON REPEAT

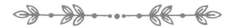

Repetition leads to habit formation. The more habitual a behavior becomes, the less cognitive effort we need to put forth, allowing us to attend to other important tasks. One way we can increase good habits is simply by doing more of the stuff that is already working rather than adding new things into the mix. It boosts confidence and is less taxing on our brains because there is no additional learning curve of a new behavior. Additionally, the more we perform a behavior that takes us closer to our goals, the more likely we are to repeat it. For this repetition to happen, we need to ensure that our environment can support this repetition and identify any deterrents that would make this difficult.

Consider a behavior you are already doing to help you achieve your goal of a healthier lifestyle (e.g., drinking more water). Rather than take on new tasks that may feel too overwhelming, such as eliminating all sugar from your diet, try increasing your daily water intake. Maybe you add in another time of day to drink water or increase your intake amount. The replication of an existing behavior can be just as effective as adding, changing or modifying another one.

On the other hand, sometimes the current frequency of behavior works just fine. An increase would not be sustainable and may set us up for failure. This exercise will help you to identify the healthy behaviors you are already doing, determine if a higher frequency would be productive, and if so, how best to sustain that increase.

In the space below provide two examples of behaviors you are already doing that are part of a habit you are trying to change or maintain.

1. ....

2. ....

For each of the behaviors you listed, offer two ways you could replicate their frequencies.

1. ....

2. ....

1. ....

2. ....

What are some potential barriers to successfully replicating your behaviors?

....

....

....

....

How can you overcome each barrier you listed above?

....

....

....

....

Based on your examples, would any behaviors allow for a sustainable increase? Why?

....

....

Which behaviors, if increased, would no longer be productive? Why?

....

....

....

Using the chart below you will track the replication of your behaviors over the course of a week. This should include any increases in frequency, duration or amount.

Habit/Pattern	SUN	MON	TUE	WED	THU	FRI	SAT
1.							
2.							
Actual time spent							

After tracking your behavior for the week, note how much time you spent in total and record your answers to the questions below.

Did you find replicating your behaviors to be easy? Why?

....

....

Did you find them to become more habitual as the week went on? Why?

....

....

Do you think choosing to replicate your behaviors was more or less effective than if you had added in a brand new behavior? Why?

....

....

Did any unforeseen barriers arise? If so, how did you resolve them?

....

....

What, if anything, would you do differently to make replication as seamless as possible going forward?

....

....

....

LESS IS MORE

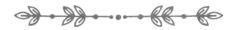

When initiating any type of behavior change, it is so important to start small and take your time. Taking on too much, too fast, can result in feelings of failure and a return to your initial unhealthy habit. When trying to reverse habits and change patterns, we often overestimate the amount we can tackle at once. It is also common to underestimate the degree to which we may fall back into old patterns, especially when under stress. Start with small goals, or what I like to call "insultingly small" goals. In other words, whatever you think you can accomplish, cut it in half. And then cut it in half again. If done properly and consistently, your behaviors will eventually become automatic and result in healthier habits. So be patient, be present, and take your time. When changing behavior, consistency is key and less is always more.

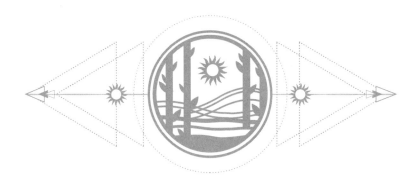

Read this scenario and then answer the following prompts:

Your visit to the doctor didn't go as planned. Your lab results suggest that your cholesterol is extremely high, you have chronic joint pain, and you are overweight. Your doctor has repeatedly told you to maintain a healthy diet, but you just can't get on board. However, after today's visit, you are starting to realize just how essential it is to change your lifestyle. Your plan is to start going to the gym five days a week for an hour every day, cook healthy food every night of the week, and cut out all soda and juice.

The next morning, you wake up at 7 am, head to the gym, and eat a healthy breakfast. That evening, you come home and cook a healthy dinner. You feel good about yourself and your accomplishments.

Day two, you wake up with a splitting headache from your sugar detox. There's no way you can go to the gym this morning; you will go after work instead. You eat your healthy breakfast and go to work. As the day winds down, you forgot that you still need to go to the gym to meet your five-times-a-week goal. But you are exhausted. You decide today will be one of your gym off days. In fact, you're too tired to cook yourself a healthy meal. You order pizza instead. Tonight will be your "free" night.

The next morning, Saturday, you wake up exhausted because you slept horribly. You think to yourself, "There is no way I can go to the gym right now. I just need to sleep." So, you sleep all through the morning of day three.

What strategies could have helped you stick to your new lifestyle change?

....

....

....

....

Now read the next scenario and answer the following prompts:

> You decide to spend your day decluttering your house. You can't
> remember the last time you sorted out your home, but it's a mess.
> Nothing is where it should be. As you look around, the idea of getting
> organized doesn't seem like such a great plan anymore. It's just too much.

In ten steps, show how you would approach this decluttering task to make it feel more possible. Remember, for behavior change to occur successfully, it is best to start slowly with "insultingly small" steps.

1. ....
2. ....
3. ....
4. ....
5. ....
6. ....
7. ....
8. ....
9. ....
10. ....

Now it's your turn. Choose a habit or behavior you wish to change or modify.

....

How would you break down the steps necessary to achieve your goal? List them here.

1. ....
2. ....
3. ....

4. ....
5. ....
6. ....
7. ....
8. ....
9. ....
10. ....

What strategies can you use to help you stick to your new lifestyle change?

....
....
....
....
....

What would it look like in six months if you were able to stick to this change?

....
....
....
....
....
....

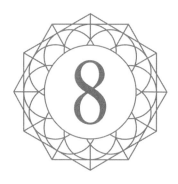

A CHAIN REACTION

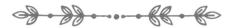

Changing habits and patterns can be exceedingly difficult and emotionally challenging. In addition to breaking things down into tiny steps, another key strategy is to link a new behavior with an existing one. For example, let's say you are working to break your perfectionistic tendencies. Part of changing these behaviors is learning to tolerate your internal discomfort when *not* engaging in them (such as resisting the urge to check and recheck the tiny details of your work so much so that you miss your deadline). A great way to learn how to sit with emotional discomfort is through grounding techniques like breathwork. If you can pair a grounding technique with an existing habit it helps to gradually introduce the new behaviors you are slowly putting into place. For example, while washing your hair in the shower you can practice a breathing exercise. Not only does this allow you to practice, but it pairs the new skill with something non-anxiety-provoking. This results in less worry and rumination in your mind, making it easier to learn new skills and information and stay on the right track.

Think of a grounding technique you would like to master:

....

....

....

....

Now, think of an everyday routine habit or behavior: one where you are typically on automatic pilot.

....

....

....

....

Over the next week, actively implement your new grounding technique during this routine task every day for one minute. After the minute is up, record your observations.

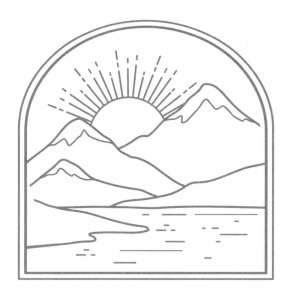

SUN

MON

TUE

WED

THURS

FRI

SAT

What came up for you during this exercise? What did you notice as your week progressed?

....

....

....

....

....

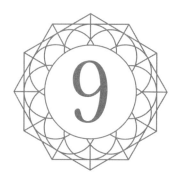

Likelihood
OF CHANGE

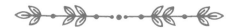

One of the most helpful strategies when changing unhealthy habits is assessing how likely you are to accomplish a new behavior. This is based on two primary factors: motivation to change and willingness to be uncomfortable.

It is so important to set small increments of change in order to develop feelings of mastery and confidence, as this is what will increase the likelihood that you will continue to make change.

If at any point a step in your path feels too overwhelming or gives you paralyzing discomfort or anxiety, simply make it smaller. You just aren't ready to tackle something that big. And that is OK. It's better to break apart the step than to avoid it altogether. Remember, consistency is more important than how much you take on.

Provide an example of a habit you wish to change. You may use the response you listed in the previous exercise, or you can use a different example. Next to your answer, give a percentage that reflects how likely you think it is that you will change this habit.

.... %

Break down the habit you wish to change into tiny behavioral components, giving each of them a percentage of likelihood that you will complete the step.

.... %
.... %
.... %
.... %
.... %
.... %
.... %
.... %
.... %
.... %

Put a star next to the component that had the lowest percentage of likelihood. Can you break that step down into even smaller components?

.... %
.... %
.... %

What do you notice now that you broke things down even further?

....
....
....

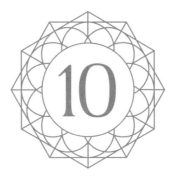

EXPOSING EMOTIONS

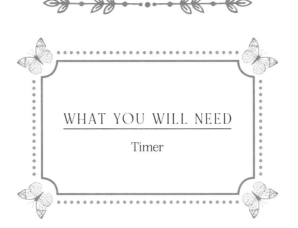

WHAT YOU WILL NEED

Timer

When we think about changing our habits, it can feel uncomfortable, overwhelming, and even scary at times. When I work with patients on changing unhealthy habits or toxic patterns, one of the most common reasons for their reluctance is the emotional discomfort they expect to have should they make the change. This is because many of our current unhealthy habits and patterns were originally formed to avoid some type of negative emotion or thought, and removing the behavior may expose this. As you go through behavior changes, it is important to identify the difficult emotions that will inevitably come with change. Noticing these emotions, acknowledging the physical sensations that may arise, and sitting with them until they pass are necessary steps for behavior change to be successful, especially for long-term maintenance. This exercise will help you identify the emotions that arise for you as you begin to change your habits and patterns.

In the space below, choose a habit or pattern that, in your opinion, is the most difficult to break.

....

....

....

....

....

....

Find a quiet spot. Close your eyes, and for sixty seconds imagine yourself in a situation where you actively change your behavior. Sit with that experience and how it feels. Notice what comes up for you during this minute.

What did you notice?

....

How did you feel?

....

What felt most difficult for you?

....

What positives do see resulting from this change?
What negatives?

....

....

....

FEEL YOUR FEELINGS

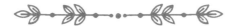

Now that you have some familiarity with how to notice and sit with uncomfortable feelings and thoughts that arise when changing behaviors, you can apply this to real-life scenarios. Record a habit or pattern below that you think would cause a mild amount of discomfort if changed. It's always best to start with something slightly uncomfortable and gradually increase over time as you become better at tolerating your discomfort.

....

....

For two weeks you are going to work on changing this. Remember, you want to start slowly and not try to tackle too much at once. Make sure your goal is clearly defined and measurable. Pay close attention to the thoughts, feelings, and bodily sensations that arise as you progress forward. Notice them as they come up and sit with them rather than trying to not have them.

For one week record your experiences below in the tracking chart. Include the target behavior, a brief description of the situation, and what came up for you in the moment.

	Behavior	Situation	Thoughts-Feelings-Emotions
SUN			
MON			
TUE			
WED			
THU			
FRI			
SAT			

After tracking your week, answer the questions below.

Did you notice any similarities across situations? (e.g., who you are with, where you are, what is going on around you):

....
....
....

What specifically were you changing? Describe what this looked like in the moment.

....
....
....

Did you notice any patterns in the thoughts, physical feelings, and emotions that came up for you?

....
....
....

Did you experience any pushback from those around you? ◯ Yes ◯ No

If yes, how did you handle the situation and what was the outcome?

....
....
....

Now that you have had time to reflect on your progress, track this habit or pattern again for another week. This time, include what changed for you in terms of your thoughts, physical feelings, and emotions compared to the last week.

	Changes in Thoughts-Feelings-Emotions	Situation	Behavior
SUN			
MON			
TUE			
WED			
THU			
FRI			
SAT			

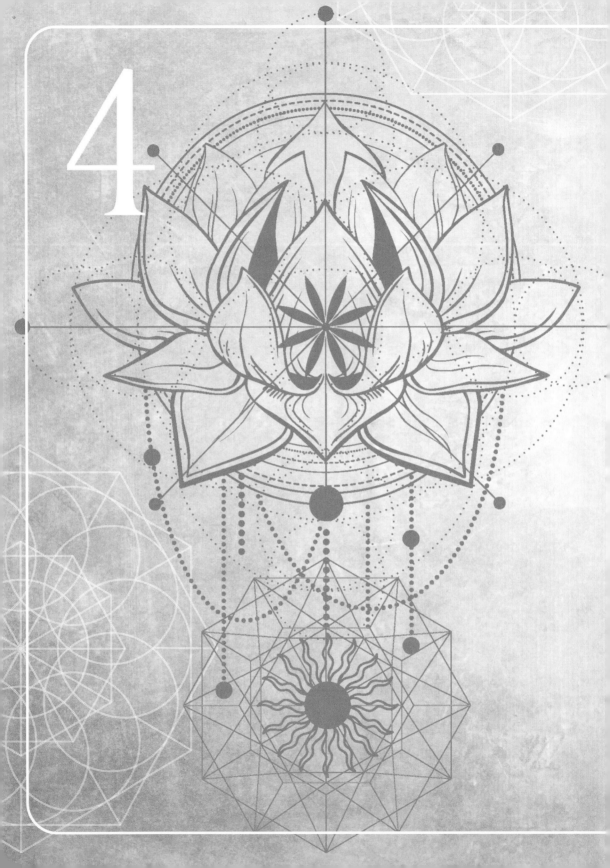

MAINTENANCE STAGE

The maintenance stage of behavior change can be the most challenging. It forces us to maintain our new behavior patterns despite barriers and obstacles that may come our way. The goal is to keep repeating the new behavior patterns until they become habitual, so that when life throws things our way, our new habits can withstand the storm.

This chapter will act as a reminder to you that we want to be continuously reassessing our patterns and habits. Are they still effective? Are they still in line with our values? Are they serving an avoidant function? Part of maintaining new habits and patterns is our willingness to be flexible and assessing if it's necessary to modify or change them.

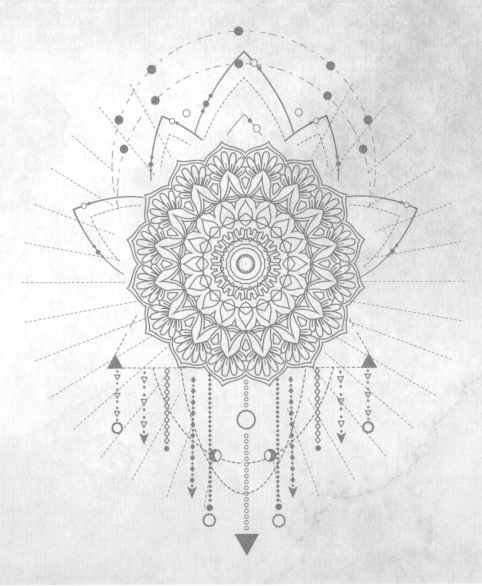

Consistency
IS KEY

The maintenance stage of behavior change can be the most challenging. It makes us maintain new behavior patterns despite obstacles that may come our way. The goal is to repeat these patterns until they become habitual, so that when life throws things our way, our new behaviors can withstand the storm.

A key aspect of this stage is consistency. The more consistent you are in maintaining new behaviors, the more comfortable they will become. Making changes in small increments keeps the reinforcement of accomplishment consistent and predictable.

How you manage a setback (or what I like to call "regrouping") is also important in this stage. Stressful situations can force our brain to take cognitive shortcuts. Setbacks may occur for all sorts of reasons, but they are quite common and, in fact, can make our progress even stronger going forward. It is important that regroupings are not viewed as failures, but as a necessary part of a lengthy process.

Another common obstacle people encounter when trying to maintain new behaviors is the response of the people around them. These are what I like to call "invisible obstacles."

Invisible obstacles are the unspoken patterns of people in your circle. This can include friend groups, family, and work. For example, let's say that you are a notorious people pleaser. You have spent much of your life taking care of everyone else's needs and have paid little attention to your own. People have grown very accustomed to you taking care of them and their emotional needs. However, after a few months in therapy, you realize that this pattern has not served you well in your adult years. So, you start to set boundaries with the people in your life; you say "no" to more things; you stop trying to always be the peacekeeper and are now putting your own needs first.

However, you are the only one within your world who is making these changes: everyone else remains the same. They are not used to you acting this way. To regain the comfortable, yet unhealthy, status quo, members of your circle will try to ease you back into your former people-pleaser role. Maintaining your new patterns in the face of these invisible obstacles can be difficult, but the more you set boundaries to protect your patterns, the easier and more habitual it will become over time.

All the World's
A STAGE

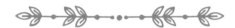

Whether you're creating new behaviors or breaking old habits and forming new ones, one of the most challenging obstacles is the people in your everyday life. Family, friends, and even colleagues are all participants in your interpersonal web, and there is a distinct dance between all these participants. That is why, when one person changes the course of their behavior, it throws the entire web off balance. To restore this balance, some people in the web will attempt to push you back to your original role. Now, this isn't necessarily intentional or malicious: it's just a normal response to something that feels "off." Others in your web, however, may have a heightened sense of awareness and are able to acknowledge your boundaries. They may not like them, but they are aware of them. There will also be people who support you in your efforts and cheer on your progress. They may even change their own behaviors for the better in response to you.

This exercise will help you map your interpersonal web and identify the unique interplay that exists within it.

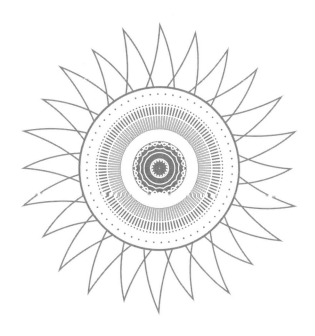

Identify all the people who you would consider part of your web. This can include immediate and extended family, friends, work colleagues, and so on.

Web Participants:

....

....

....

....

....

....

....

....

....

In the space below, map out your participants in relation to you, with you in the center of your web.

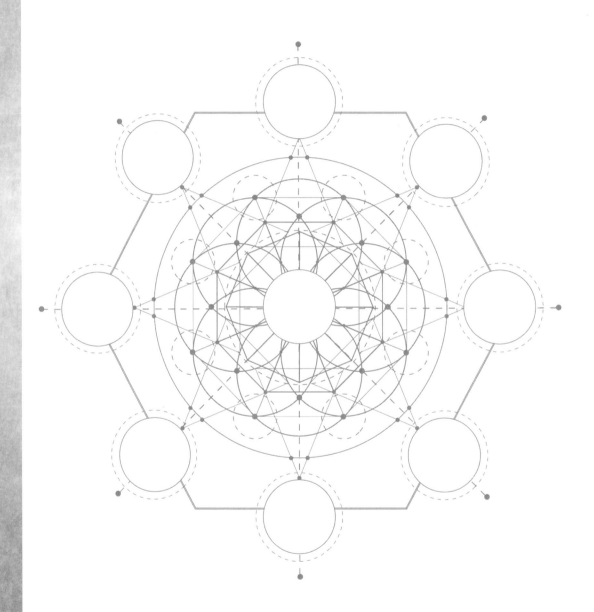

Pick one habit or pattern that you wish to change or improve upon and record
it below.

....

....

If you were to initiate that change right now, how would those in your web respond
to you? Would your behavior change impact how they respond to each other?
In the space below, write a brief description of each person's response to your
new behavior.

....

....

....

....

....

....

....

For example, let's say you want to reduce time spent on your phone because it has
become all-consuming. How would changing this habit impact your relationship with
your mother? Maybe she would be concerned that she can't reach you immediately
like she used to. So she calls your father repeatedly to express her worry. Your
father then calls you, pleading with you to answer your phone when your mother
calls. This is an invisible obstacle.

The function of your dad's plea is to restore balance, to push you back into
your previous role (phone obsessed) so everyone can go back to normal. Even in
this simple example, you can see how one small behavior change has impacted
two people in your web. Sometimes just the tiniest shift in behavior can be
very empowering.

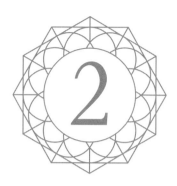

Overcoming
OBSTACLES

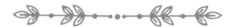

Maintaining positive habits and patterns can be challenging at times. Mental health issues, lack of social support, work, financial difficulties, and even everyday stress can present as obstacles to long-term maintenance of these healthy patterns. It is unrealistic to assume that we can avoid all obstacles that may jeopardize our behavior changes. However, by identifying them early on, we can be better prepared to deal with them when they do arise.

This exercise will help you identify potential barriers and obstacles you may encounter during the maintenance phase of change.

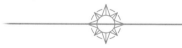

In the space below, write down a habit you would like to change or a pattern you would like to modify. You may use one from a previous exercise, if you like.

Below, list any obstacles or barriers that could impact your ability to maintain healthy behavior change in the future. The more detailed you are with your responses, the easier it will be to develop an effective plan.

1. ....
2. ....
3. ....
4. ....
5. ....

What would be an effective strategy to help you maintain your new behaviors if confronted with the obstacles listed above? For example, let's say you want to be less of a perfectionist. You identify "work project deadlines" as an obstacle. You know from previous experience that your perfectionism significantly interferes with your ability to meet deadlines. An effective strategy could be simply breaking down the project into smaller components. This will make the project seem less daunting and overwhelming and allow you to develop that sense of accomplishment early on. Another example is quitting drinking. Let's say you haven't had a drink for three months, but the holiday season is approaching and you've been invited to a party. This time of year could certainly be viewed as an obstacle, and formulating a plan ahead of time would be beneficial. Maybe you ask the host to not serve alcohol, maybe you commit to staying for a shorter period of time, or maybe you have friends and family you can contact for support during dinner.

Provide one strategy for each obstacle you've listed.

1. ....
2. ....
3. ....
4. ....
5. ....

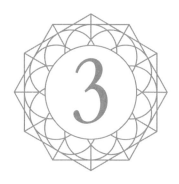

Remember
THE ROUTINE

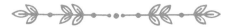

Maintaining newly implemented habits and patterns requires increased levels of awareness, focus, and attention. To be able to sustain this degree of cognitive effort, we must first possess the means to do so. Daily routines are extremely effective strategies to conserve cognitive energy. Examples of routines may include the order in which you get yourself out the door to work each morning, your workout schedule, the steps you take when showering, or even the manner in which you grocery shop. Routines allow us to predict what comes next, limit unnecessary stress, and free up brain space so we can attend to other things in our lives. The more routines we implement, the more attentional resources we have available to focus on maintaining new behaviors.

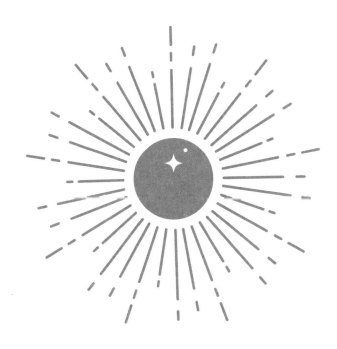

What routines do you currently have in your daily life that make your day-to-day easier?

....

....

....

....

In what other areas of your life could you implement a routine to make your day-to-day easier?

....

....

....

....

For each area you listed above, describe the routine you would choose to implement.

Area of life: ....

....

....

....

....

How does implementing this routine make your life easier?

....

....

....

....

Area of life: ....

....

....

....

....

How does implementing this routine make your life easier?

....

....

....

....

Area of life: ....

....

....

....

....

How does implementing this routine make your life easier?

....

....

....

....

Area of life: ....

....

....

....

....

How does implementing this routine make your life easier?

....

....

....

....

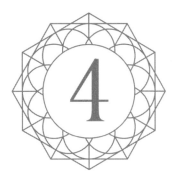

The Impossibility
OF INCONSISTENCY

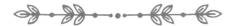

Think about a salaried job: every two weeks, you're paid a set amount of money. You know what your job description is, what your projected performance measures are, and what is expected of you. Should your job description ever change, you are given significant notice to adjust effectively to your new role. How much anxiety would you expect to have about your biweekly paycheck? Probably very little.

What if, however, not only are you not informed of your job description and what is expected of you, but you are never told when you'll be paid or how much. Sometimes you're paid $400 on Monday, $50 on Friday, and nothing for the next three weeks. And just when you think you've figured out the schedule, everything changes again. How much anxiety would this cause for you? Probably a significant amount.

This is because of something known as "intermittent reinforcement." It creates that feeling of never knowing what you're going to get and having little control over your external environment. As you can imagine, this type of reinforcement leads to heightened anxiety and significantly lower goal achievement. It is so important that when changing habits or patterns, you establish a consistent and predictable environment.

For the examples on the next page, record if the scenario would either help or hurt you to maintain a new habit.

You have been working hard to improve your sleep patterns. You get into bed at the same time every night, turn off all electronics an hour before bed, and have limited your caffeine intake.

To maintain healthy sleep, you remain vigilant about your diet during the day, limiting caffeine and carbohydrate consumption. You and your roommate split daily living tasks, and they are responsible for the food shopping.

Will this help you maintain your healthy sleep pattern? ....

Why? ....

You decide to limit your sugar intake prior to bed and start with no sugars after 6 pm for three nights per week.

Will this help you maintain your healthy sleep pattern? ....

Why? ....

Your significant other has been a night owl most of their life. They usually stay up late playing video games with their friends and drinking energy drinks, rarely going to sleep before 1 am. To help maintain your healthy sleep hygiene, you ask your partner to come to bed by 10 pm.

Will this help you maintain your healthy sleep pattern? ....

Why? ....

You are going to implement a workout routine two mornings a week. Your roommate has agreed to join you, which is great, because you don't have your own car to get to the gym.

Will this help you maintain your healthy sleep pattern? ....

Why? ....

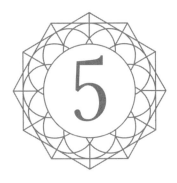

Take Control
OF THE CHAOS

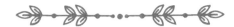

The more control we have over how we maintain our behaviors, the more likely we are to be successful. In the examples you considered in the previous exercise (see page 130), for those that you thought wouldn't help you maintain your new sleep hygiene habits, think of an alternative that would give you more control over your environment and behavior maintenance.

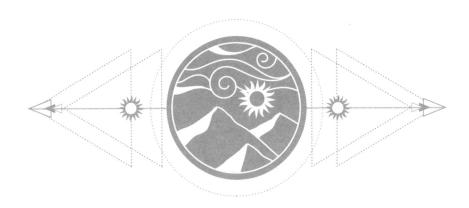

1. ....

....

....

2. ....

....

....

3. ....

....

....

In your own life, what do you notice when you alter your environment to have more control over your circumstances?

....

....

....

Think about three areas of your life in which you are actively changing patterns and behaviors. It could be your alcohol intake, study routines, dating behavior, or even family relationships.

1. ....

2. ....

3. ....

For each of your examples above, list something that feels out of your control and provide an alternative strategy that increases the likelihood of continued maintenance.

1. This is out of my control:

....

I'll have more control if:

....

....

2. This is out of my control:

....

I'll have more control if:

....

....

3. This is out of my control:

....

I'll have more control if:

....

....

Over the next week, implement these modifications in an effort to gain more control over your environment, then record your experiences below:

What did you find most difficult about trying to gain control over your environment?

....

....

....

Were there certain areas that were easier to control than others?
Why do you think this was the case?

....

....

....

Did you notice any type of pushback from the people around you?

....

....

....

Did these efforts for control lead to improved maintenance? Why?

....

....

....

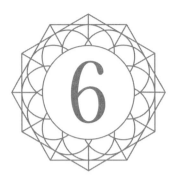

Becoming BOUNDARIED

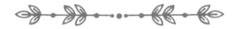

What are boundaries? Boundaries are any action, or inaction, that lets those around you know what you are willing to accept or not, and how you are willing to be treated. Boundary setting is a key component in changing relationship patterns.

Maybe *the* most important fact about boundaries is this: They are for YOU and only YOU. We have no control over how others will respond to our boundaries. All we can do is maintain them by being as consistent as possible. Inconsistent boundaries can be highly detrimental to maintaining pattern and habit change. Consistency allows us to walk away feeling more in control and more likely to engage in that healthier pattern again.

Below, list a few boundaries you have set or tried with others in the past. This could be choosing not to text someone back right away, blocking someone on social media, or saying "no" to taking on more work.

1. ....
....
....

2. ....
....
....

3. ....
....
....

4. ....
....
....

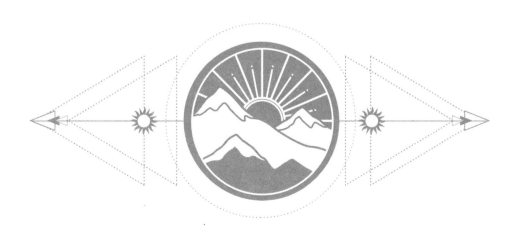

A key part of boundary setting is: Only set a boundary if you think you are able to maintain it consistently. Inconsistent boundaries can lead to more of the behavior you don't want. They send mixed signals to others and create a vicious cycle of confusion, toxic behaviors, and heightened emotions. For example, say you recently got out of a long-term relationship. Despite your repeated requests to your ex-partner that they stop contacting you, they disregard your wishes completely, and then when they message you, you respond; you respond because you don't want to appear rude or mean.

It is very difficult to maintain your boundaries because when you set them you feel a sense of guilt. In your effort to not feel guilty, you end up creating the exact cycle you are trying to avoid. Sometimes you text back and other times you don't. This intermittent responding creates *more* of the undesirable behavior (texts from your ex) and increases the feeling of guilt you are trying so hard to avoid. If, however, you could sit with your guilty feelings *and* not respond to their messages, these feelings would dissipate over time. And, eventually, the messages from your ex will as well.

My patients often tell me that they set a boundary but it didn't work. However, it isn't that their boundary failed, it's that they based its success on the other person's response. It is important to remember that setting boundaries is for *you*. They are a way to let others know what you're willing to tolerate and how you wish to be treated. Boundary setting is *not* for the other person. We have no control over their behaviors; we can only control how we respond to them.

In the spaces below, provide an inconsistent alternative to each of the four boundary examples you gave above.

1. ....
....

2. ....
....

3. ....
....

4. ....
....

For each of the four boundary examples you gave above, describe what you think would happen if you implemented the boundary inconsistently.

1. ....
....

2. ....
....

3. ....
....

4. ....
....

What emotions and thoughts do these bring up for you?

....
....

PUSH PULL

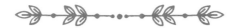

Just as you have a pattern of relating to others, they have one with you. What happens when you change your pattern, even ever so slightly, and the other person does not? What if *you* are the only one with the awareness, willingness, and motivation to change? This is often the case when I work with patients. It is quite common for people to seek therapy when their interpersonal relationships are stressed, whether by work, marital conflicts, dating difficulties, or family discord. Therapy often focuses on identifying these relational patterns and acknowledging those that work and those that don't. However, by changing your behavior, you throw the entire system off balance. As we discussed earlier, everyone in your relationship web has a role, and when you alter your steps, you mess up the dance.

So, what can this look like? Imagine having been a people pleaser for as long as you can remember. Your primary concerns have centered around taking care of others' needs before your own, fearing that if you make yourself a priority, this would make you selfish. Maybe you didn't feel deserving of having your needs met. Or maybe you feared others would get angry with you or dislike you. However, after working hard on changing your patterns, you begin to set boundaries.

Think about how those around you might respond to your new behavior patterns. Will they be accepting? Will they say you're being selfish? Get angry at you? What would they say to push you back into your original people-pleaser role?

Your new pattern: ....

....

Their response: ....

....

Your new pattern: ....

....

Their response: ....

....

Your new pattern: ....

....

Their response: ....

....

What did you observe while coming up with these examples?

....

....

Did it feel uncomfortable to imagine yourself following this new pattern?...................

If yes, why?...

....

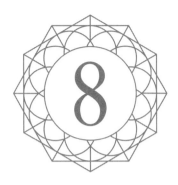

Pushback
TO THE PUSHBACK

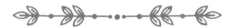

When it comes to relationships, it can be difficult to maintain
your boundaries and/or new patterns of interacting.

Having identified anticipated responses from others in the previous exercise,
what are some ways you can continue to maintain your behavior changes
despite the sometimes inevitable pushback you may receive? For example,
what if a new pattern of saying "no" to your mother is met with her saying,
"Why are you so selfish?" How can you respond and still maintain your
healthy pattern? Again, keep in mind that inconsistency in your pattern-
setting will not only lead to heightened negative emotions, but also make it
even harder to make healthy change going forward.

....

....

....

....

....

....

When you have attempted setting ongoing boundaries in real life, did you find that you became more or less anxious?

....

Was there a particular person or situation that made it more uncomfortable for you?

....

....

What was most anxiety-provoking for you?

....

....

What thoughts or fears were going through your mind as you committed to maintaining your pattern?

....

....

Would it have been easier in the moment to just go back to your old patterns?

....

What would have happened if you did just that?

....

....

Chances are, you might have felt a temporary relief of anxiety or fear by resorting back to old patterns, but this avoidance of discomfort would be short-lived.

Pitfalls
AND TRIGGERS

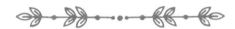

A key component of maintaining new habits and behaviors is identifying ahead of time anything that may make it difficult to keep yourself on the right track. Think about habits (such as biting your nails) or patterns of behavior (such as chronic lateness) that you wish to work on and list them below, alongside any pitfalls or triggers you anticipate that could get in your way.

Habit/Pattern: ....

Pitfalls/Triggers:

....

....

Habit/Pattern: ....

Pitfalls/Triggers:

....

....

Habit/Pattern: ....

Pitfalls/Triggers:

....

....

When becoming more aware of triggers and pitfalls, it is helpful to track them in the moment. As they show up for you in your day-to-day life, keep a record of what they are and the situations in which they occur. This will help you to not only become more aware of your triggers, but also their frequency and in what context they arise. You may record them in the chart below. As you track your triggers and pitfalls over time, try to notice any patterns or themes that emerge. For example, are there certain situations that your triggers show up more frequently? Do your triggers seem to all relate to one another? Do your pitfalls all occur at a particular time during the day?

	Trigger/Pitfall	Date & Time	Context it occurred
SUN			
MON			
TUE			
WED			
THU			
FRI			
SAT			

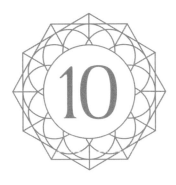

If at First You DON'T SUCCEED...

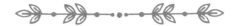

It's easy to forget that behavior and habit changes are a process. They are not a one-and-done fix. Pattern change is often fluid, meaning our approach to situations will shift and change over time as we change along with our contexts. You will mess up. You will make mistakes. It is inevitable. Believe it or not, learning from our mistakes is a necessary component of maintaining healthy changes. We learn what works and what doesn't, when it works, and with whom it works best. Take trading on the stock market, for example. There is a pattern to trading. Stick with the pattern, and you can typically manage your losses. However, there are times when one deviates from the working plan; you may feel it in your gut, you may be very sure of yourself, but you end up losing money in the trade. You allowed your emotions to get the best of you. So, what do you do now? Throw your hands up and walk away because you failed? Continue to make risky trades to regain your losses? Or do you take a pause, regroup, and get back on the track that you know works? Learning how to take a pause, reset, and regroup after messing up is just as important as setting the healthy behavior in the first place.

Using the spaces on the next page, think of a few instances in which you messed up, got sidetracked, or resorted to older, unhealthier habits or patterns.

1. ....

2. ....

Did these setbacks impact your perception of yourself and
your ability to change unhealthy behaviors?
How so?
◯ Yes   ◯ No

....

....

How did you handle the negative thoughts and emotions that came up for you?

....

....

Approximately how long did it take you to get back on track and what strategies
did you use?

....

....

Using the strategies you have learned in this workbook, what would you do differently?
Would you have handled your setbacks in another way?

1. ....

2. ....

What preventative measures could you implement to decrease the chances of getting
off track again in the future?

1. ....

2. ....

Control
WHAT YOU CREATE

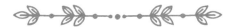

In addition to identifying potential roadblocks to maintaining new habits and patterns, it is also important to ensure that your current environment is able to support you. In other words, do you have everything you need set in place before initiating behavior changes? Think about what would be necessary to make this change process as seamless as possible. Do you require a support system? A therapist? Alcohol and drug support groups? Or maybe you require more tangible items, such as finances, a gratitude journal, a behavior tracking app, or a gym membership? What about a recent physical with your primary care doctor or medication?

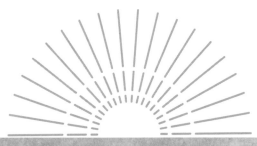

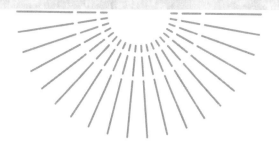

In the space below, list two unhealthy habits. They don't need to be personal examples.

1. ....
2. ....

For each of the above habits, make a list of all the things you would need to create an environment that supports your efforts.

1. ....   1. ....
2. ....   2. ....
3. ....   3. ....
4. ....   4. ....
5. ....   5. ....
6. ....   6. ....

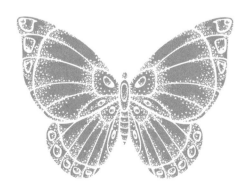

Remember
THE WHY

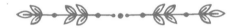

We are not perfect. We will make mistakes. In fact, attempts to be perfect can often lead to increased anxiety and a regression to unhealthy patterns. Not only does maintaining healthy change involve modifying our behaviors as needed, but it also involves what I like to call a "reassessment of benefits."

Every now and again, it is important to take a pause and assess our relationships, behaviors, and mental well-being. During this "reassessment of benefits," it is imperative that we ask ourselves if our current habits and patterns are still as effective as they once were. Are they continuing to help us live the healthiest version of ourselves or do they need modification based on life changes? Remember, patterns are fluid. Even ones that you worked so hard to implement may eventually need a tune-up. As discussed in the beginning of this workbook, avoiding necessary behavior change can lead to a whole host of emotional, physical, and relational difficulties. These reassessments of benefits serve as reminders of *why* this change was so important to you in the first place.

What are some behavior changes you have made or unhealthy habits you have broken? You may use examples from the previous exercises. Underneath each example, conduct a reassessment of benefits. In other words, what is your *why?* *Why* did you want to change this behavior in the first place? How did you anticipate that this change would impact your well-being and relationships?

Change made/habit broken:

....

....

Reassessment of benefits:

....

....

Change made/habit broken:

....

....

Reassessment of benefits:

....

....

Change made/habit broken:

....

....

Reassessment of benefits:

....

....

CONCLUSION

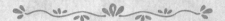

It is my hope that this workbook has given you a fundamental understanding of how to change unhealthy patterns and habits. Behavior change does not occur overnight. It is a long and uncomfortable process. Breaking a habit can take a considerable amount of time. Learning your triggers, tolerating the discomfort of not doing the behavior, and maintaining your progress over time is hard work. Pattern change is a constantly evolving process that involves flexibility and adaptation, without which people will often report feeling "stuck"— stuck in relationships, families, and in their careers. This feeling of being trapped is typically the result of unhealthy and ineffective behavioral patterns. While people can identify feeling stuck or unhappy in their lives, they have more difficulty gaining awareness of how their own behavioral patterns influence their life choices.

As we now know, not all patterns and habits are bad. In fact, most are extremely helpful in our daily lives. Habits provide us with routine, a sense of mastery and control within our environment. Healthy patterns offer us a playbook of sorts. They make us feel safe in unfamiliar situations and are the foundation upon which we interact with other people. In addition, patterns and habits allow our brains to work more effectively and help us to not become easily overwhelmed. When we engage in habitual behaviors, our brains can switch onto automatic pilot and direct our attentional resources to newer, more unfamiliar information in our environment.

Patterns of behavior are often longstanding, having originated in childhood. They have a very specific and adaptive function: to help the child navigate their world. The child is able to rely on these patterns to make sense of their environment and relationships. As the child gets older and their world expands, it is expected that their patterns will adjust accordingly to accommodate their new experiences. However, when patterns do not evolve over time, they stop making sense within the person's world. Once patterns stop serving an adaptive purpose, people will begin to feel increasingly more unfulfilled in their lives. What once worked for them as a child has become maladaptive, and the longer they maintain these unhelpful patterns, the more at risk they become for stress, relationship issues, anxiety, depression, and substance abuse.

Letting go of the familiar can be a scary process, especially when changing longstanding habits and patterns. Difficult feelings can come up and negative self-talk emerges. Changing behaviors involves motivation, flexible thinking, and a willingness to change despite the emotional discomfort that may come up during this process. It's important to learn ways to tolerate these feelings in the moment yet still move forward toward your goals, and that avoiding discomfort will only lead to the repetition of unhealthy behaviors.

Change does not always come easy. Accepting that it may feel bad at times and that messing up is part of the change process will help you establish appropriate and realistic goals. You are likely working against years of repetition and familiarity, so be sure to manage your expectations. Allow for mistakes, setbacks, and imperfections. Remember that what is healthy for one person may not be healthy for another. Be gentle with yourself. Be patient. If you do the hard work, healthy change will follow.

REFERENCES

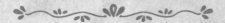

Harris, Russ. *The Reality Slap: Finding Peace and Fulfillment When Life Hurts.* Oakland, CA: New Harbinger Publications, Inc., 2012.

Hayes, Steven C. *A Liberated Mind: How to Pivot Toward What Matters.* New York: Avery Publishing Group, 2020.

Hayes, Steven C. and Smith, Spencer. *Get Out of Your Mind and Into Your Life: The New Acceptance and Commitment Therapy.* Oakland, CA: New Harbinger Publications, Inc., 2005.

Mckay, Matthew, Wood, Jeffery C., and Brantley, Jeffery. *The Dialectical Behavior Therapy Skills Workbook: Practical DBT Exercises for Learning Mindfulness, Interpersonal Effectiveness, Emotion Regulation, and Distress Tolerance,* 2nd Edition. Oakland, CA: New Harbinger Publications, Inc., 2019.

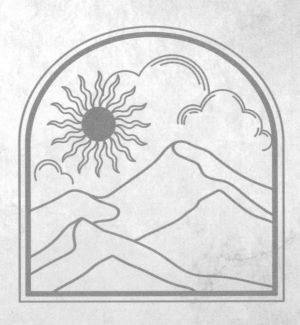

RESOURCES

Anxiety. American Psychological Association, https://www.apa.org/topics/anxiety

"Anxiety Disorders." National Alliance on Mental Illness, https://www.nami.org/About-Mental-Illness/Mental-Health-Conditions/Anxiety-Disorders

Bacow, Terri. *Goodbye, Anxiety: A Guided Journal For Overcoming Worry.* Seattle: Spruce Books, 2021.

Forsyth, John P., and Eifert, Georg H. *The Mindfulness and Acceptance Workbook for Anxiety: A Guide to Breaking Free from Anxiety, Phobias, and Worry Using Acceptance and Commitment Therapy,* 2nd Edition. Oakland, CA: New Harbinger Publications, 2016.

Harris, Russ. *ACT Made Simple: An Easy-to-Read Primer on Acceptance and Commitment Therapy,* 2nd Edition. Oakland, CA: New Harbinger Publications, 2019.

Hayes, Steven C. and Smith, Spencer. *Get Out of Your Mind and Into Your Life: The New Acceptance and Commitment Therapy.* Oakland, CA: New Harbinger Publications, Inc., 2005.

Meditation Minis, https://meditationminis.com/

ShrinkChicks Podcast, https://podcasts.apple.com/us/podcast/shrinkchicks/id1483261668

The Anxiety Coaches Podcast with Gina Ryan, https://podcasts.apple.com/us/podcast/the-anxiety-coaches-podcast/id908153168

ACKNOWLEDGMENTS

I would like to thank Quarto for presenting me with another opportunity to write a workbook. Thank you to my editors, Katie Moore and Elizabeth You, for their continued patience and guidance. As always, a heartfelt thank you to my brilliant colleagues, Drs. Jen Wolkin and Rachel Goldman, for their expertise, support, and friendship. And a special thank you to my amazing administrative assistant, Sophia Liss, who literally holds my life together.

To all my professors, supervisors, and mentors over the years, thank you for continuing to influence me in my work. I would like to acknowledge the groundbreaking work of Drs. Steven Hayes, Kelly Wilson, Aaron Beck, Zindel Segal, Mark Williams, John Teasdale, and Marsha Linehan. Their evidence-based theories are the framework of this workbook.

Lastly, I want to express my gratitude to all my friends and family. Without any of you, none of this would be possible. Thank you for constantly motivating and supporting me during this journey.

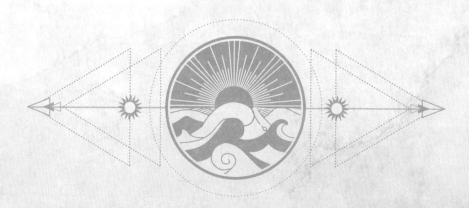

ABOUT THE AUTHOR

Dr. Jaime Zuckerman is a graduate of the Ohio State University and obtained her doctorate in clinical psychology from La Salle University. She trained at various Philadelphia-area hospitals, including Temple University and the University of Pennsylvania's prestigious Center for Cognitive Therapy. She completed both her predoctoral internship and postdoctoral training at Long Island Jewish Medical Center in Queens, New York. Dr. Z is a licensed clinical psychologist in private practice outside Philadelphia. She practices both Cognitive Behavioral Therapy and Acceptance and Commitment Therapy in the treatment of anxiety and mood disorders in adults. Dr. Z also specializes in narcissistic abuse and offers coaching services for those involved in narcissistic relationships.

Dr. Z is a mental health social media influencer and media contributor. She has been featured in various publications including *Vogue, Insider,* the *Harvard Business Review, Women's Health,* and the *Washington Post,* with an Ask the Expert column in *Verywell Health.* Dr. Z is a frequent guest expert on various podcasts and news outlets, including

Fox29 News, PHL 17, CBS3 Philly, Daily Mail TV, and The List TV. Additionally, she is co-host of the podcast "It's Me, Dr. Z with JB" and author of *Find Your Calm: A Workbook to Manage Anxiety.*

Dr. Z is a professional board member of the Epilepsy Foundation of Eastern Pennsylvania (EFEPA) and is a frequent conference presenter for both the EFEPA and the Dravet Syndrome Foundation. Dr. Z lives in the suburbs of Philadelphia with her husband and three children. When not working/reading/writing/speaking/posting and momming, she loves playing tennis, reading psychological thrillers, and watching documentaries.

For additional mental health resources, including virtual workshops, social media, videos, article features, and TV appearance links, please see the links and social media handles below:

Website: www.drjaimezuckerman.com
Podcast: "It's Me, Dr. Z with JB," available on Apple Podcasts or wherever you listen to your podcasts
Instagram: @dr.z_psychologist
Twitter: @drzpsychologist
TikTok: @dr.z_psychologist
YouTube: Dr. Jaime Zuckerman
Facebook: @drjaimespinellzuckerman

NOTES